RENAL AND UROLOGIC DISORDERS

NEPHROLITHIASIS

RISK FACTORS, TREATMENT AND PREVENTION

Renal and Urologic Disorders

Additional books in this series can be found on Nova's website under the Series tab.

Additional e-books in this series can be found on Nova's website under the e-book tab.

RENAL AND UROLOGIC DISORDERS

NEPHROLITHIASIS

RISK FACTORS, TREATMENT AND PREVENTION

MELODY SHNEIDER
EDITOR

New York

Library of Congress Cataloging-in-Publication Data

ISBN: 978-1-63482-134-6
Library of Congress Control Number: 2015931172

Published by Nova Science Publishers, Inc. † New York

Contents

Preface

Nephrolithiasis is the third most common diagnosis involving the urinary tract, exceeded only by urinary tract infections and prostate conditions. Uric acid nephrolithiasis accounts for 5–10 % of all kidney stones in the general population in the United States (US) and is noted to be increasing in other parts of the world like Japan, previously known to have a low incidence of this condition. This increase is attributable, at least in part, to westernized eating habits. Other factors which influence development of kidney stones include age, sex and ethnicity. This book discusses in further details, the risk factors, treatment options and ways to prevent nephrolithiasis.

Chapter I – Urinary calculi (nephrolithiasis) is the third most common diagnosis involving the urinary tract, exceeded only by urinary tract infections and prostate conditions. It is a common condition with an annual incidence of 0.5% to 1.0%. Prevalence in the U.S. has been increasing from 3.8% to 8.8% in the period 2007-2010, with a lifetime risk of 13% for men and 7% for women. Factors which influence development of kidney stones include age, sex, ethnicity as well as the geographical area. The risk of nephrolithiasis is influenced by urine composition. Infections, genetic defects, metabolic and anatomic factors, and certain drugs can increase the risk of stones. Risk factors vary according to the type of stone. Obesity, a diet high in animal protein, increased salt intake, and oxalate-containing foods are associated with the formation of calcium oxalate stones. Poor urinary drainage or indwelling catheters increase risk for urinary tract infections and struvite stones. Uric acid stones are associated with acidic urine, which is more common in obese patients with metabolic syndrome and insulin resistance, or in patients with chronic diarrhea. Calcium phosphate and calcium oxalate stones share some risk factors such as low urine volume, high urine calcium, and low urine citrate. Despite the identification of these risk factors formation of the majority of stones is idiopathic and understanding of their underlying mechanism of formation remains speculative. Patient education remains the key method of preventing stone formation. Patients must be instructed to drink at least 2 to 3 liters of water daily. The common misconception that a low calcium diet can reduce the risk of kidney stones must be debunked and patients should be taught that adequate intake of dietary calcium actually can prevent stone formation. People with nephrolithiasis should undergo evaluation to identify risk factors and precipitating events so that appropriate measures can be taken to prevent future stone development. Management of this condition ranges from conservative treatment with pain medication and hydration until passage of the stone to urgent urologic consultation in patients with urosepsis, acute renal failure, anuria, or dehydration. Stones not passed spontaneously or with medical expulsive therapy can be treated with extracorporeal lithotripsy, or removed via ureteroscopy. Large stones may require percutaneous nephrolithotomy (PCNL) or open surgery. The treatment choice depends on a multitude of factors including location of the stone, magnitude of the obstruction, stone composition, function of the affected and unaffected kidneys, presence or absence of urinary tract infection, advancement of stone passage, and surgical risk of the individual patient. Half of patients with a first calcium-containing stone have a recurrence within 10 years. Twenty-five percent of struvite stones relapse if there is incomplete removal of the stone. Fortunately, the percentage of nephrolithiasis-related end-stage renal disease (ESRD) appears small (3.2%) and long-term complications of kidney stones are infrequent. In this review we will further elucidate the risk factors which precipitate nephrolithiasis as well as provide an overview of preventive and treatment strategies of this common disorder.

Chapter II – Uric acid nephrolithiasis accounts for 5–10 % of all kidney stones in the general population in the United States (US) and is noted to be increasing in other parts of the world like Japan, previously known to have a low incidence of this condition. This increase is attributable, at least in part, to westernized eating habits. The prevalence of uric acid nephrolithiasis has continued to rise at alarming rates in high risk populations, such as patients with type 2 diabetes mellitus, obesity and metabolic syndrome. In these conditions, there are changes in the serum and urine chemistries leading to more acidic urine and chronically increased uric acid production, which are both pre-requisites for the formation of uric acid stones. The clinical presentation is similar to any other kidney stone that includes pain radiating from the flank into the pelvic area, as the stone moves downward, and concomitant associated symptoms such as nausea, vomiting, fever and hematuria can be also present. These stones are diagnosed by CT as plain x-rays are not helpful since uric acid stones are not radiopaque. The treatment for uric acid stones is well-defined nowadays; consisting of alkalinizing the urine and increasing fluid intake, and in selected cases, the use of xanthine oxidase inhibitors might be needed. In this review, we focus on the pathophysiology diagnoses, causes, treatment and prevention of uric acid stones.

Chapter III – *Purpose:* The aim of this review is to examine the utility of ureteroscopy in the management of ureteral stones. *Introduction:* Throughout ureteroscopy's relatively brief history, clinical utility has paralleled technological advancement. This review follows that progression beginning with Dr. Young's placement of a pediatric cystoscope into a child's dilated ureter. *Technique:* The method for both rigid and flexible ureteroscopy is discussed. We will also review potential pitfalls and discuss techniques that can help avoid potential complications. Finally, the debate on the use of ureteral stents during ureteroscopy is examined. *Results:* Although the efficacy of ureteroscopy is well documented, this review pays particular attention to factors which influence stone free rates and how to maximize success. Risk factors for complications are identified and techniques proposed to achieve the highest possible success rates based on expert experience. *Discussion:* Ureteroscopy is a safe and effective option for management of ureteral stones. Using the techniques described here, stone free rates are extremely high and risk is minimized. Furthermore, with the decreasing size of ureteroscopic instruments and improving images, complication rates should continue to decline.

Chapter IV – The incidence of calcium stones is increasing world-wide. Dietary changes which impact on urine composition are probably largely responsible. However, despite years of research, we still do not have a clear understanding of the underlying defects in hypercalciuria or hyperuricosuria in idiopathic calcium stone formers or of how diet is implicated. Without this, interventions to prevent stone recurrence are largely empirical and often biased by personal opinion. From the authors' stone clinic they reported that male stone formers with idiopathic hypercalciuria reabsorb less of the calcium filtered into the kidneys than men with normocalciuria. Similarly, net urate reabsorption of men with idiopathic hyperuricosuria is reduced compared with those with normal urate excretion. This is probably explained by genetic variation in the renal transport of calcium and urate in the general population. In an earlier study, in which the authors investigated families in which three or more first degree relatives had stones, they confirmed the heritability of hypercalciuria. From our growing knowledge of the numerous genes which are implicated in the renal handling of calcium and urate, and of their close interaction, genetic variation is inevitable. There is increasing interest in this area, but so far few associations have been identified between genetic polymorphisms of renal transporters and hypercalciuria or hyperuricosuria. From their clinic, the authors also found subsets of male stone formers with hypercalciuria and hyperuricosuria who had very high creatinine clearance rates, and hence (by inference) glomerular filtration rates. This would lead to delivery of an abnormally high filtered load of calcium or urate to the kidneys. They do not know the explanation. However, one possibility is a high dietary protein intake. There is a large body of evidence that high intakes increase glomerular filtration. From recent studies this might be mediated by enhanced nitric oxide production via the renal arginine-citrulline cycle, which could also influence intrarenal blood flow. This merits further exploration. As in the case of hypercholesterolemia, idiopathic hypercalciuria and uricosuria may result from interaction between increased genetic susceptibility and dietary excesses, particularly of protein. Whilst identification of those with unfavorable diets and appropriate intervention should reduce calcium or urate excretion of hypercalciuric and hyperuricosuric stone formers, it will not be enough for those at the more severe end of the spectrum for genetic abnormality. They will need additional medication which, hopefully, may be targeted towards specific transporters in the future. With the advances in the technology for rapid through-put DNA analysis, we now have the opportunity to get to the roots of the problem, but it will be fundamental to define the phenotypes of stone formers as precisely as possible if the genetic analyses are to be fruitful.

Chapter V – Lithiasis of the urinary tract is nowadays recognized as a significant health care issue, affecting millions of people worldwide and resulting in hospital admissions, medication prescription, elaborate surgical treatment and loss of working hours. Although major advances and innovations have taken place in the field of active stone management, there is little progress in the field of preventative measures. Recurrent stone formers, i.e., patients who most likely suffer from metabolic stone disease, are particularly affected, as practices vary amongst physicians and institutions. In this chapter, we shall attempt to look into a risk factor-oriented approach to the contemporary preventative strategies in urolithiasis. Following a preliminary introduction into the epidemiology and pathogenesis of the disease, the authors shall present an individualized strategy for the various categories of metabolic and non metabolic stone formers, in a coherent and systematic fashion. They shall outline the importance of an integrated metabolic stone unit in tertiary care centers, by describing the structure and function of a state-of-the-art unit and also emphasize on desirable outcomes.

Chapter VI – Nephrolithiasis is an important manifestation of autosomal dominant polycystic kidney disease (ADPKD), which ranges from 8% to 36% in different studies. It is a frequent cause of morbidity because of flank pain, hematuria, and urinary tract infections. Nephrolithiasis is as common in females as in males and is asymptomatic in 50% of patients. Half of polycystic kidney disease patients are symptomatic and 20% require surgical removal of the stones. The etiology of stone disease in ADPKD is multifactorial, including both anatomic abnormalities (large, obstructing cysts and dilated tubular lumens may create tubular stasis, which predisposes to stone formation) and metabolic factors (hypocytraturia, hyperuricosuria, hyperuricemia and low urine pH). Also, in this high frequency contribute some risk factors such socioeconomic status of patients, geographic zones and dietary habits (most of them were from rural areas, consuming less water, more vegetable and animal proteins). Patients with a larger kidney volume predominant cyst size are at a higher risk of stone formation. Because of patients with ADPKD have a frequent occurrence of renal calcifications, the CT scan provides an excellent technique for detecting calcifications and for distinguishing renal calculi from cyst calcifications in patients with ADPKD. In ADPKD patients, the principles of management of kidney stones are the same as in patients with normal kidneys: percutaneous nephrolithotomy, while shock wave lithotripsy and open surgery are only indicated on few conditions. After removal of kidney stones, risk factors evaluation and control should always be considered to prevent or to reduce the frequency of recurrent stone disease in such patients.

Chapter VII - Up to one-third of the patients with Autosomal Dominant Polycystic Kidney Disease (ADPKD) develop nephrolithiasis; this prevalence is seven to ten-fold higher as compared to the general population. Additionally, morbidity related to stones is especially high in ADPKD – nearly half of the patients with nephrolithiasis have symptoms over the course of their lifetime and one-fifth of the symptomatic patients require urological intervention. Risk factors for stone formation in ADPKD are both structural and metabolic. In particular, more than half of the stones are of uric acid composition. With normal urate handling observed in this group, this propensity for uric acid crystallization is attributable to increased urinary acidification and lower urinary pH seen in ADPKD. One mechanism that may explain this finding is the stimulatory effect of an overactive renin-angiotensin-aldosterone-system, a consequence of local parenchymal ischemia from compression by expanding cysts on the α-intercalated cells in the collecting duct system. Although most surgical techniques, including extracorporeal shock wave lithotripsy and percutaneous nephrolithotomy, are effective in stone removal, the risks of complications and residual stones are higher in ADPKD as compared to those in the non-ADPKD population with nephrolithiasis. A high rate of stone recurrence underlines the importance of dietary and medical management for secondary stone prevention in this population. Clinical evaluation, including a 24-hour urine metabolic profile, is needed to determine the precise risk factors in an individual patient and for developing the appropriate strategy for minimizing future stones. Our focus is on the various aspects of stone disease unique to ADPKD, including the reasons for high incidence of stones (in particular, uric acid stones); the nuances of diagnosis, evaluation and treatment unique to this population; and the different strategies for secondary prevention in affected patients.

In: Nephrolithiasis
Editor: Melody Shneider
ISBN: 978-1-63482-134-6

Chapter I

An Overview of Nephrolithiasis Risk Factors, Prevention and Management

Monica C. Chiang, MD, Taniya N. De Silva, MD, and Gabriel I. Uwaifo, MD.

Section of Endocrinology, Diabetes and Metabolism, Department of Medicine; LSU Health Sciences Center-New Orleans, LA, US

Abstract

Urinary calculi (nephrolithiasis) is the third most common diagnosis involving the urinary tract, exceeded only by urinary tract infections and prostate conditions. It is a common condition with an annual incidence of 0.5% to 1.0%. Prevalence in the U.S. has been increasing from 3.8% to 8.8% in the period 2007-2010, with a lifetime risk of 13% for men and 7% for women. Factors which influence development of kidney stones include age, sex, ethnicity as well as the geographical area.

The risk of nephrolithiasis is influenced by urine composition. Infections, genetic defects, metabolic and anatomic factors, and certain drugs can increase the risk of stones. Risk factors vary according to the type of stone. Obesity, a diet high in animal protein, increased salt intake, and oxalate-containing foods are associated with the formation of calcium oxalate stones. Poor urinary drainage or indwelling catheters increase risk for urinary tract infections and struvite stones. Uric acid stones are associated with acidic urine, which is more common in obese patients with metabolic syndrome and insulin resistance, or in patients with chronic diarrhea. Calcium phosphate and calcium oxalate stones share some risk factors such as low urine volume, high urine calcium, and low urine citrate. Despite the identification of these risk factors formation of the majority of stones is idiopathic and understanding of their underlying mechanism of formation remains speculative.

Patient education remains the key method of preventing stone formation. Patients must be instructed to drink at least 2 to 3 liters of water daily. The common misconception that a low calcium diet can reduce the risk of kidney stones must be debunked and patients should be taught that adequate intake of dietary calcium actually can prevent stone formation. People with nephrolithiasis should undergo evaluation to identify risk factors and precipitating events so that appropriate measures can be taken to prevent future stone development.

Management of this condition ranges from conservative treatment with pain medication and hydration until passage of the stone to urgent urologic consultation in patients with urosepsis, acute renal failure, anuria, or dehydration. Stones not passed spontaneously or with medical expulsive therapy can be treated with extracorporeal lithotripsy, or removed via ureteroscopy. Large stones may require percutaneous nephrolithotomy (PCNL) or open surgery. The treatment choice depends on a multitude of factors including location of the stone, magnitude of the obstruction, stone composition, function of the affected and unaffected kidneys, presence or absence of urinary tract infection, advancement of stone passage, and surgical risk of the individual patient. Half of patients with a first calcium-containing stone have a recurrence within 10 years. Twenty-five percent of struvite stones relapse if there is incomplete removal of the stone. Fortunately, the percentage of nephrolithiasis-related end-stage renal disease (ESRD) appears small (3.2%) and long-term complications of kidney stones are infrequent.

In this review we will further elucidate the risk factors which precipitate nephrolithiasis as well as provide an overview of preventive and treatment strategies of this common disorder.

Introduction

Nephrolithiasis also known as kidney stones or urinary calculi is a common disorder with an increasing incidence and prevalence worldwide over the past 20 years. Currently in industrialized countries the prevalence has been estimated as 6% in women and 12% in men but these rates continue to rise. [1]

In the United States, the National Health and Nutritional Examination Survey (NHANES) noted a prevalence of nephrolithiasis of 8.8% during the period from 2007 to 2010. This marked a significant increase when compared to the prevalence of 3.8% reported in the period from 1976-1980. [2] This increase in prevalence was noted in all age, gender, and racial-ethnic groups particularly in black and Hispanic populations.

Kidney stones account for significant morbidity and frequent hospitalizations thereby leading to high economic costs. Nephrolithiasis has been associated with chronic kidney disease that can progress to end stage renal disease (ESRD) and thus with significant risk for subsequent cardiovascular events. [2-4]

Kidney stones form when urine becomes oversaturated. Factors that can lead to oversaturation include those that affect chemical free ion activity including the urinary ion concentration, urinary PH, and precipitation induced by other substances. When chemical free ion activities are increased the urine becomes oversaturated leading to the formation of new stones or growth of established stones. In a setting of decreased free ion activity, urine may become undersaturated. In this setting stones do not grow and in fact may even dissolve.

The composition of kidney stones may vary. Calcium oxalate comprises about three fourths of all stones, calcium phosphate (7%), uric acid (5%), magnesium ammonium phosphate (struvite 10 to 20%) and cysteine (less than 1%). [2,5] The type of stone formed is dependent on a number of pathogenic mechanisms.

Risk Factors

There are several factors that impact the prevalence and incidence of stone formation, including gender, age, race, geographic distribution, sunlight exposure and urinary composition. Both patient habits and genetic predisposition can influence these risk factors.

Clinically the lithogenic potential of the urine is evaluated by measuring the rates of excretion of the principal stone-forming elements.

Hypercalciuria is an excessive urinary calcium excretion. Hypercalciuria can be defined in many ways. However, each definition has its limitations.

Hypercalciuria can be defined as a urinary calcium excretion greater than 300 mg/day in men and 250 mg/day in women. No clear explanation exists as to why men tolerate a higher calcium load in the urine than women. However there is substantial variability in the cut off points utilized for urinary calcium excretion amongst both research and clinical laboratories with some using the same cut off for both males and females. For example, alternative definitions of hypercalciuria include urinary calcium excretion of calcium greater than 200 mg/day or greater than 4 mg/kg per day. The main weakness of such references values lie in the fact that the risk of stone formation below these cut offs with calcium excretion above 100 mg/day is still considerable. [6]

The major contributors to increase in urinary calcium excretion include increased bone resorption (resorptive hypercalciuria), increased intestinal absorption (absorptive hypercalciuria), [7] and increased renal loss (renal hypercalciuria) characterized by a defect in calcium reabsorption at the level of the renal tubules. Most patients with hypercalciuria have more than one underlying defect contributing to their increased urinary calcium levels.

High urine calcium excretion without an identifiable cause is referred to as idiopathic hypercalciuria and is considered the most common cause of calcium containing kidney stones. [8] This is a polygenetic familial disorder initially thought to be transmitted in autosomal dominant pattern.

There are many other genetic causes of hypercalciuria. Genetic causes of kidney stones secondary to increased bone resorption include multiple endocrine neoplasia type 1 (MEN1), McCune Albright Syndrome, infantile hypophosphatemia, and osteogenesis imperfecta type 1. Conditions resulting in hypercalciuria due to increased intestinal absorption include congenital lactate deficiency, Down's syndrome and hypophosphatemia. Disorders linked to renal hypercalciuria include Dent's Disease, Bartter's syndrome, and familial hypomagnesemia with hypercalciuria and nephrocalcinosis (FHHNC). [9-14]

Nephrocalcinosis is an extensive deposition of calcium phosphate or calcium oxalate in the kidney parenchyma (cortex and/or medulla). The crystalline deposition can be at either molecular, microscopic or macroscopic with the latter being the form typically detected clinically by findings on radiologic imaging. This condition may be seen with normal renal function but predisposes the development of acute or chronic kidney injury. Nephrocalcinosis may be diagnosed incidentally by imaging studies performed for other reasons not related to renal pathology. The prognosis of patients with this condition is dependent on the underlying cause. Those patients with nephrocalcinosis due to FHHNC or Dent's disease (X linked recessive nephrolithiasis) are more prone to develop end stage renal disease (ESRD). No specific management has been shown to prevent progression of nephrocalcinosis. The exact factors that cause some patients to develop nephrocalcinosis instead of or in addition to nephrolithiasis are still poorly understood.

Hyperoxaluria is an increase in oxalate excretion. [14] Oxalate is primarily produced through the endogenous metabolism of glycine and ascorbic acid. Elevations in urinary oxalate may be secondary to increased dietary intake of certain types of food, including beets, spinach, rhubarb, strawberries, nuts, chocolate or beans. [15,16] Absorbed oxalate is excreted unchanged in the urine. The consequent supersaturation of the urine is an augmented risk for stone formation. The standard definition of normal urinary oxalate excretion is less than 45 mg/day. However, even oxalate excretion levels above 25 mg/day enhance the risk of stone formation significantly. [6,17]

The three major causes of hyperoxaluria are excessive oxalate ingestion (dietary oxaluria), malabsorptive gastrointestinal disorders (enteric oxaluria) and excessive endogenous production of oxalate associated with a hepatic enzyme deficiency (primary hyperoxaluria).

Oxalate absorption is affected by calcium in the gut by formation of insoluble calcium oxalate salts in the intestinal lumen as the formation of these salts results in decreased oxalate absorption and leads to reduced oxalate excretion in the urine. This is an important concept for kidney stone management. A similar concept applies in absorptive hyperoxaluria where malabsorbed fatty acids bind calcium in the intestinal lumen, making more free oxalate available for absorption. [18,19]

Gastrointestinal flora can impact the metabolism of oxalate. For example, the bacterium oxalobacter formines stimulates the degradation of oxalate and enteric excretion of oxalate thereby leading to decreased oxalate excretion in the urine. [20-22] The potential clinical benefit of this is under investigation. The administration of antibiotics can lead to alterations in gastrointestinal flora, which can affect oxalate metabolism and thereby increase the risk of stone formation.

Primary hyperoxaluria is a genetic disorder which results in massive endogenous oxalate production secondary to hepatic enzyme deficiencies. This condition results in both hyperoxaluria and the widespread deposition of oxalate in different organs and tissue. [23]

High doses of vitamin C may result in increased oxalate generation as a result of the metabolism of ascorbic acid. It has been estimated that urinary oxalate excretion increases 6 to 13 mg/day for every 1000 mg of vitamin C ingested above 500 mg/day. [24]

Hyperuricosuria is an increase in the urinary uric acid concentration. The mechanism by which uric acid excretion predisposes to calcium stone formation is unclear. Statistical reports estimate that 15% of calcium stones occur in patients with hyperuricosuria. [5,25] Support for the role of hyperuricosuria in calcium stone formation comes from a randomized controlled trial in which allopurinol significantly reduced the likelihood of calcium oxalate stone recurrence in calcium stone formers with hyperuricosuria but normal urinary calcium excretion. [4]

Hypocitraturia is defined as a urinary citrate level below 320 mg/day. This cut off point is also controversial as it has been described that men tend to have lower urinary citrate concentration than women. [6] Citrate combines with calcium to form a soluble complex that reduces precipitation of calcium phosphate and calcium oxalate. Additionally, it appears to inhibit the process of crystal agglomeration. Therefore, citrate is considered an important protective inhibitor of kidney stone formation. [26-29]

Metabolic acidosis is an important inhibitory factor of citrate excretion in urine. Acidosis leads to calcium and phosphate release from bone as well as rise in proximal tubular reabsorption of citrate and reduced tubular reabsorption of calcium.

When citrate is absorbed from the gastrointestinal tract, a small amount is not metabolized by the liver. This unmetabolized citrate leads to increased blood citrate and increased renal citrate excretion. [30] This occurs whether citrate is ingested as citric acid or as citrate salt. Citrate salt ingestion causes systemic alkalinization, which decreases renal citrate reabsorption and increases urine citrate excretion.

Citrate excretion is dependent more on the extent of systemic alkalinization than on the direct delivery of unmetabolized citrate to the kidney. As a result, any compound that causes a systemic alkalosis increases citrate excretion. Malate is a polycarboxylic anion, like citrate, that is present in many fruit juices and carbonated beverages. If delivered as an alkali salt, malate can also increase urinary citrate. [31]

Inhibitors of stone formation present in normal urine include glycoproteins such as Tamm-Horsfall mucoprotein, nephrocalcin and uropontin. [32-34]

It is well known that calcium phosphate and calcium oxalate stones share some risk factors such as low urine volume, high urine calcium, and low urine citrate. Hyperoxaluria is a risk factor for calcium oxalate stones while higher urine pH is a risk factor for calcium phosphate stones. Because the approach to stone prevention depends on the composition of the stone, it is essential that every attempt is made to retrieve a passed or removed stone and to send it for analysis.

Risk factors for stone formations can be stratified according to stone composition. [35-37]

	Calcium Stone	Uric acid Stone	Struvite Stone	Cystine Stone
Urinary Risk Factors				
Hypercalciuria	+			
Hyperoxaluria	+			
Hyperuricosuria	+	+		
Hypocitraturia	+			
Low urinary volume	+	+	+	+
Urinary pH		<5.5	>6.5	<5.5
Recurrent urinary infections	+		+	
Dietary Factors				
High animal protein intake	+	+		+
Inadequate fluid intake	+	+	+	+
High sodium intake	+			
High fructose and sucrose intake	+	+		
Other Medical conditions				
Obesity	+	+		
Metabolic Syndrome	+	+		
Malabsorption	+	+		
Cushing's Syndrome	+	+		
Gout	+	+		
Diabetes Mellitus	+	+		
Medications				
Acetazolamide	+			
Topiramate	+			
Loop diuretics	+			
Allopurinol		+		
Salicylate		+		
Theophylline	+			
Probenecid		+		
Genetic disorders				
Cystinuria				+
Glucose 6 phosphate deficiency	+	+		
Lesch Nyhan Syndrome	+	+		
Multiple Endocrine Neoplasia Type 1 (MEN1)	+			
McCune Albright Syndrome	+			
Infantile Hypophosphatemia	+			
Osteogenesis Imperfecta Type 1	+			
Down Syndrome	+			
Dent's Disease	+			
Bartter's Syndrome	+			
Primary Hyperoxaluria	+			
Familial Hypomagnesemia with hypercalciuria and nephrocalcinosis (FHHNC)	+			
Hereditary Hyperphosphatemic Rickets with Hypercalciuria	+			
RTA type 1 (due to hereditary causes)	+			

Figure 1. Risk factors associated with kidney stone formation.

Major Factors Associated with CALCIUM Stone Formation

- **Urinary risk factors:**

Hypercalciuria: (Cushing's syndrome, granulomatous diseases, hypercalcemic disorders, idiopathic hypercalciuria, immobilization, malignancy, milk alkali syndrome, primary hyperparathyroidism, sarcoid and thyrotoxicosis)

Hyperoxaluria: (Biliary obstruction, chronic pancreatitis, Crohn's disease, dietary and enteric oxaluria, jejunoilial bypass, malabsorptive disorders, bariatric surgery, large doses of vitamin C)

Hypocitraturia: (Androgens, exercise, hypokalemia, hypomagnesaemia, infections, metabolic acidosis, starvation)

Hyperuricosuria (see below)

- **Dietary risk factors:**

High oxalate intake
High animal protein intake
High sodium intake
Low fluid intake
High sucrose and fructose intake
High vitamin C intake (especially in men) leading to hyperoxaluria

- **Anatomic risk factors:**

Medullary sponge kidney
Horseshoe kidney
Tubular ectasia
Congenital megacalix

- **Other medical conditions:**

Gout
Obesity
Diabetes Mellitus
Renal Tubular Acidosis type 1

- **Medications:**

Acetazolamide
Amphotericin B
Topiramate
Antacids
Glucocorticoids
Loop diuretics
Theophilline
Vitamin C – (producing hyperoxaluria)

Vitamin D
Laxatives

Major Factors Associated with URIC ACID Stone Formation

- **Urinary risk factors: [35,36]**
  Low urine pHh <5.5
  Low urine volume
  Hyperuricosuria (Gout, Cushing's syndrome, glucose 6 phosphate deficiency, diarrhea, excessive insensible losses, hemolytic anemia, inborn error of metabolism, Lesch-Nyhan Syndrome, malabsortive disorders, tumor lysis syndrome, myeloproliferative dissorders
- **Dietary risk factors:**
  High animal protein intake
  Excessive dietary purine intake
  Inadequate fluid intake
- **Other medical conditions:**
  Obesity
  Insulin resistance leading to diabetes mellitus
  Cushing's syndrome
  Metabolic syndrome
  Genetic predisposition
- **Medications:**
  Allopurinol
  Probenecid
  Salicylates

Major Factors Associated with STRUVITE (magnesium ammonium phosphate) Stone Formation

- Urease producing bacteria (proteus, pseudomonas, haemophilus, yersinia, ureaplasma, klebsiella, corynebacterium, serratia, citrobacter, staphylococcus, others)
- High urine pH
- Indwelling urinary catheter
- Neurogenic bladder

Major Factors Associated with CYSTINE Stone Formation

- Autosomal recessive trait
- Excessive excretion of cystine, ornithine, lysine and arginine
- Low solubility of cystine

Other Considerations That Increase the Risk of Stone Formation

Patients with a family history of stones have a greater than two fold increased risk of stone formation. [38] This in part is due to the many genetic and hereditary disorders that constitute risk factors for stone formation.

Nephrolithiasis is associated with a recurrence rate of 14% within 1 year in patients with a first kidney stone. The percentage increase to 35% within 5 years with higher incidence in men than women. [39]

Medications that can crystallize in the urine include IV acyclovir, indinavir, nelfenavir, sulfonamides, triamterene, and prolonged ceftriaxone therapy. [35,36,40-42]

Occupation can be relevant to stone formation. People engaged in fields such as surgery or jobs involving frequent travel often minimize fluid intake to avoid frequent micturition throughout the day. This places them at risk of stone formation. Other professions or hobbies such as construction, gardening and running can expose people to an increased loss of insensible fluid, which decrease urinary output and predispose to stone formation.

The quality of fluid ingested can also contribute to stone formation though the data on this subject is sometimes conflicting. Consumption of sugar-sweetened beverages is associated with an increased risk of developing kidney stones. [43] In contrast, prospective studies reveal that increased tea and coffee consumption have been associated with a lower risk of stone formation. Alcoholic beverages have been shown in some studies to increase the risk of stones. However, other studies have noted a lower risk of stone formation with consumption of beer and wine. [43-45] Orange juice (which contains both potassium and citrate) as well as several sodas rich in citrate were associated with a lower risk of crystal formation most likely due to increased urinary citrate excretion. [46-48]

History of ingestion of herbal preparations and supplements has to be taken into considerations as potential risk factors for stone formation. [49]

Risk Factors by Special Groups

The increase in prevalence of diabetes, obesity and hypertension in children has been associated with an increase of kidney stones in children, particularly among adolescents. [50 51,52] Kidney stones in children are more likely to be related to anatomic and metabolic abnormalities, increased urinary calcium excretion, decreased urinary oxalate and citrate excretion, and much higher urinary calcium oxalate saturations than children with no history of kidney stones. [50,51]

During pregnancy there is an increase in the glomerular filtration rate associated with a higher urinary calcium excretion. In the second and third trimesters there is also an increase in the urinary pH. These physiologic changes are considered predisposing factors for calcium phosphate stone formation. It is reported that pregnant women are twice as likely to have calcium phosphate stone compared with non-pregnant women. They are two to three times more likely to have calcium phosphate stones than oxalate stones. [53] Kidney stones during pregnancy increase the risk of urinary tract infections and preterm delivery. [54]

Obesity is a well-known epidemic problem in the United States and worldwide. As per the (NHANES), the measured prevalence of obesity in adults in the United States is currently estimated at approximately 34.9 percent. [55] Previous studies have demonstrated that obesity can increase the risk of stone formation as well as recurrence rates of stone disease. Recent studies have shown obesity to be associated with unique changes in serum and urinary chemistry studies such as increased urinary excretion of calcium, citrate, sulfate, phosphate, oxalate, uric acid and cystine. [56] Several studies cite an increased risk of nephrolithiasis among obese patients. [4,44,57,58] An inverse relationship between BMI and urine pH has been described.

Obesity is associated with a high rate of recurrent stone formation. The etiology of this association is multifactorial. Obese patients often consume a diet high in animal proteins. They have increased risk of diabetes mellitus and hyperuricemia both of which can increase the risk of stone formation. Obese patients should undergo a targeted metabolic evaluation to evaluate for stone risk. Dietary counseling for obese patients should include recommendations regarding intake of animal protein. In these patients, therapy with allopurinol (xanthine oxidase inhibitor), can be useful as it both decreases urate production and urate excretion in the urine. Potassium citrate is an alternative therapy to treat hyperuricosuria. Together, careful metabolic evaluation, dietary counseling and pharmacologic therapy can significantly decrease the risk of recurrent stone formation in obese patients. [59]

Prevention

Prevention of kidney stone formation is based upon decreasing the concentrations of lithogenic factors such as calcium and oxalate and increasing the concentrations of inhibitory factors of stone formation, such as citrate. This target can be achieved via dietary modification and pharmacologic therapy.

Current evidence is insufficient to conclude that an assessment of baseline stone composition, blood chemistry, or urine chemistry prior to the initiation of pharmacologic therapy or dietary interventions reduces stone recurrence. [60]

Most patients, irrespective of stone type, are given general advice about fluid and dietary modifications to prevent further stone formation. It is well known that higher fluid intake reduces the risk of incident and recurrent kidney stones. Increased fluid intake reduces recurrent kidney stones by approximately 40% reduction over 5 years. [44,45,61]

Dietary Modifications

Increase Fluid Intake

Patients should be advised to increase fluid intake to raise urine volume to approximately 2 to 2.5 liters per day with special attention paid to the types of beverages consumed.

Grapefruit juice may be associated with an increased risk of stones, especially calcium oxalate stones. The potential lithogenic factor in grapefruit juice has not yet been elucidated.

Coffee, and tea have been reported in prospective observational studies to be associated with a lower risk of stone formation. Caffeine has been reported to increase diuresis moderately. It has also been shown to increase the excretion of magnesium, potassium, calcium and sodium.

Cranberry juice is well known to be used as prophylaxis against recurrent urinary tract infections. However, when ingested in large amounts cranberry juice increases the urinary saturation of calcium oxalate. [62] While ingestion of moderate amounts of cranberry juice is unlikely to be harmful there is no evidence that this beverage is beneficial for stone prevention.

Orange juice is rich in potassium citrate, and it favorably affects urine composition and risk of stone formation by increasing citraturia. [48,63]

There are multiple observational studies regarding soda intake and potential benefits and harms associated with its content. Higher consumption of sugar-sweetened soda was associated with a higher incidence of kidney stones, because of its fructose content. Fructose increases the urinary excretion of calcium, oxalate, and uric acid, therefore increase the risk of stones formation. [64-66] On the other hand, several commonly consumed diet sodas contain high amounts of citrate in the form of alkali, malate as alkali and total alkali (in amounts even higher than a lemonade beverage commonly used for hypocitraturic nephrolithiasis). These beverages may be helpful for dietary treatment for hypocitraturia. Further studies are necessary to discern whether these findings would have beneficial clinical effects. [67]

Limit Sodium Intake

Patients are counseled to limit the daily sodium intake to a maximum of 3000 mg/day (130 meq/day) in an attempt to reduce hypercalciuria. Dietary sodium restriction decreases urinary sodium and reduces calcium excretion by enhancing proximal sodium and calcium reabsorption. [68]

Reduce Animal Protein Intake

It is recommended to reduce moderately animal protein ingestion to approximately 1.0 mg/kg/day. Dietary animal protein generates a mild metabolic acidosis that increases urinary calcium excretion and reduces urinary citrate excretion. The metabolism of sulfur-containing amino acids increases the generation of sulfate ions, which couple with calcium ions to form insoluble complexes. Dietary protein may also lead to increased calcitriol production. The metabolism of purines leads to an increased generation of uric acid. Animal protein is much more likely to induce this effect than vegetable protein since it has a higher sulfur content and therefore, generates more acid. [69] Multiple studies have reported that a diet high in animal protein is a risk factor for stone formation in men but not in women. [69,70] A reduction in animal protein intake does produce changes in urine composition but has not been proven to reduce the incidence of stone formation. [71,72]

Increase Fruit and Vegetable Intake

It is established that withdrawing fruits and vegetables from the diet of healthy subjects decrease the urinary excretion of potassium, magnesium, citrate, and oxalate, as well as increase the urinary excretion of calcium and ammonium. Such changes are contributing factors for stone formation. [73] Fruits and vegetables are rich in potassium; hypokalemia can lead to reduce citrate excretion and may increase the risk of calcium oxalate stone formation. Therefore, an increase in potassium supplementation can be a useful strategy in the prevention of kidney stones.

Increase Potassium Intake

Data suggests that a diet rich in potassium can result in a substantial reduction in the risk of stone formation. [74] This is due to the fact that potassium-rich foods tend to have a high alkali content, and this elevated alkali concentration can result in a decreased urinary calcium excretion and increased urinary citrate excretion. Fruit and vegetables are the main sources of dietary potassium.

Limit Sucrose and Fructose Intake

Fructose consumption has markedly increased over the past decades. It is an omnipresent sweetener in American processed food. The mechanisms underlying the relation between fructose, and stone risk are unknown, but may be related to the effect of fructose intake on urine composition. It is believed that fructose intake increases the urinary excretion of calcium as well as increases the endogenous generation of oxalate and uric acid. Studies have proven that fructose intake is positively and independently associated with an increased risk of nephrolithiasis. [66]

Sucrose intake has also been associated with an increased risk of stone formation in younger and older women. High oral glucose intake has been linked to an increase in urine calcium excretion. [75,76]

Limit Dietary Oxalate Intake

There is scant evidence that low oxalate diets reduce the risk of stone formation. [51] Some foods traditionally believed to be high in oxalate, such as tea, do not increase the risk of stone formation. Therefore, low oxalate diet should only be continued if there is documented evidence that implementation of the diet has led to a decrease in urine oxalate excretion.

Patients with dietary hyperoxaluria should be provided with a list of high oxalate foods. How restrictive the patient should be is unknown, especially as many patients with a history of kidney stones also have hypertension, diabetes mellitus and would consequently benefit from a diet that is high in fruits and vegetables.

Calcium Intake

Dietary calcium restriction is no longer recommended unless urinary calcium is greater than 2000 mg/d.

As the majority of stones contain calcium and since hypercalciuria has been associated with the formation of stones, calcium restriction has been routinely recommended for patients who have kidney stones. Many studies have proven that a low calcium diet has long-term efficacy in reducing calcium excretion and may influence the risk of stone formation. [68,74]

However, as a low calcium diet generates low levels of calcium in the intestinal lumen following this diet can lead a decrease in calcium bound oxalate. Decreasing the oxalate bound by calcium can lead to an increase in urinary oxalate excretion and urinary saturation. [68] In fact, calcium restriction increases the absorption of oxalate in the gastrointestinal tract in normal subjects and in patients with kidney stones, leading to an increase of 16% to 56% in urinary oxalate excretion. [74]

Data comparing utilization of low calcium diets versus normal calcium diets in the prevention of stone formation, reveals that due to a net increased oversaturation of the urine with respect to calcium oxalate low calcium diets actually can predispose patients to stone formation. [68,75] In addition, dairy products may be a source of some other, as yet not identified, protective factor. [77]

Quantity of dietary calcium is not an independent variable; gender, age, use of calcium supplements, time of administration of supplements, and kind of supplement utilized all appears to play important roles in altering the risk of stone formation. Patients should be advised to maintain an age and gender appropriate intake of dietary calcium preferably without supplements. [77]

A low calcium diet may have additional deleterious effects in patients with idiopathic hypercalciuria. Patients on low calcium diets may develop a negative calcium balance with consequent loss of bone density. In some patients, this occurs as a result of bone resorption stimulated by PTH secretion. [9,78,79] In patients with concomitant osteoporosis and nephrolithiasis the risks and benefits of dietary calcium supplementation should be carefully weighed.

Phytate

Phytate is a well known inhibitor of calcium oxalate crystal formation in vitro. [75] It is believed that phytate forms insoluble complexes with calcium in the intestinal lumen and reduces calcium absorption and urinary calcium excretion, which subsequently may reduce the risk of stone formation. Dietary sources of phytate include cold cereal, dark bread, and beans. [77]

Management

There are many possible treatment options for nephrolithiasis. Optimal management strategies vary based upon stone location, size, and composition, the presence or absence of patient comorbidities and available surgical expertise. In septic patients, emergent therapy is utilized to decompress the collecting system to relieve symptoms, decompress the collecting system and to avoid potential imminent complications. [80]

Although location of stone is important stone size is the major determinant of the likelihood of spontaneous stone passage. Stones smaller than 5 mm in largest diameter have a 68% chance of passing spontaneously, while those larger than 5 mm have a spontaneous passing rate of 50%. [80] Most stones greater than 10 mm, and many of those between 5 and 10 mm in size, will require surgical intervention. Therefore the management of kidney stones can be divided into those requiring medical versus surgical therapy.

Medical Therapy

Patients with acute renal colic can be managed conservatively with pain medication and hydration, especially in those individuals with a newly diagnosed ureteral stone less than 10 mm in greatest diameter. Observation with periodic evaluation should be continued until passage of the stone. Medical expulsive therapy (MET) is an option for patients with well-controlled pain, no clinical evidence of sepsis, and adequate renal functional reserve. Several medications have demonstrated benefit in reducing the time to stone passage and in assisting with passage of larger stones.

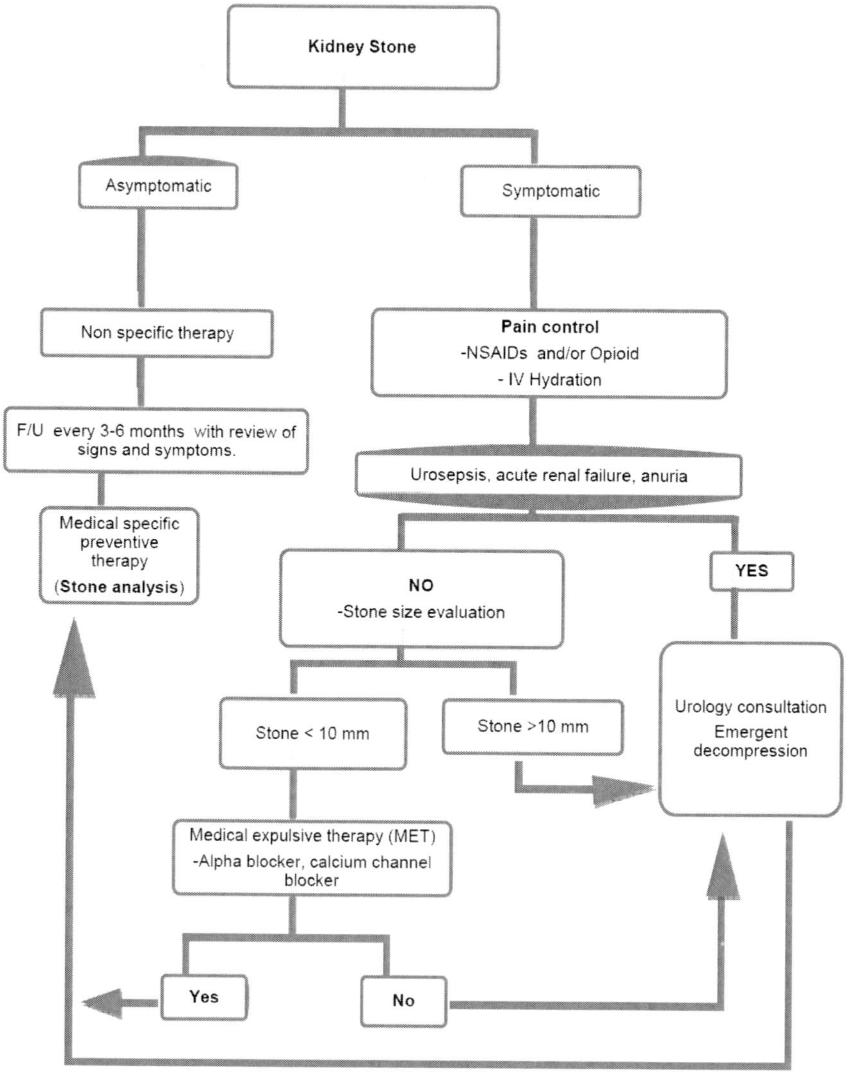

Figure 2. Algorithm of management for kidney stones.

Pain Control

Aggressive hydration with an increase in fluid intake and oral analgesic are recommended. Patient can be managed as outpatients if they are able to tolerate oral intake. Nonsteroidal anti-inflammatory drugs (NSAIDs) in combination with narcotics (opioids) is the preferred treatment of renal colic. NSAIDs act by direct inhibition of ureteral smooth-muscle contraction at the site of the obstructing stone, and by alleviating of the renal capsular distention caused by vasospasm of the afferent arterioles. [81,82] Data suggests than some NSAIDs can be as effective as opiates for pain control, with higher rates of nausea, vomiting, and dizziness noted in patients treated with opioids. [81-83] NSAIDs use can also lead to greater reduction in pain scores. Patients treated with NSAIDs are also less likely to require further analgesia in the short term. Use of algorithms favoring NSAIDs use rather than narcotics also discourages opiate-seeking patients from fabricating symptoms of renal colic. [83] Use of NSAIDs however, can result in acute kidney injury particularly in patients with dehydration and preexisting kidney disease. Therefore, combination of therapy with NSAIDs and opioids has been reported to be superior to either agent alone.

Facilitating Stone Passage

In animal models, ureteral stones result in an increased amplitude of ureteral smooth-muscle contraction, a decreased frequency of contractions, and decreased ureteral pressure. [84] Evidence suggests that relaxation of the ureter in the region of the stone and concomitant increase of hydrostatic pressure proximal to the stone can help to facilitate ureteral stone passage. [85] Relaxation can be accomplished through the administration of adrenergic α-antagonists and calcium-channel blockers. The effects of these drugs are mediated respectively through the calcium-channel pumps and adrenergic α-1 receptors present in ureteral smooth muscle. [86,87] Randomized controlled trial indicate that patients treated medically with calcium-channel blockers or α-blockers had a 65% greater likelihood of spontaneous stone passage when compared to patients not given these drugs. [88] The use of alpha blockers may be superior to calcium channel blockers with studies noting faster stone passage, fewer hospitalizations and procedures, and less hypotension inpatients treated with alpha blockers. [88] Based on this data treatment with tamsulosin 0.4 mg daily is recommended to facilitate spontaneous stone passage in patients with stones $\leq$10 mm in diameter. The addition of corticosteroids may also assist with stone passage by reducing local ureteral inflammation and swelling at the site of the stone. Concurrent antibiotics therapy has been used by some groups. However, there is currently no supporting data available to validate this practice. Though effective for stone expulsion treatment with medications for MET carries with it the potential side effects of hypotension, palpitations, and headaches.

MET may be attempted for 4 to 6 weeks as long as pain is well controlled, the patient has normal or stable kidney function, there is no evidence of urinary tract infection, and the patient does not have either a solitary obstructed kidney or bilateral obstruction. Careful monitoring and follow up with intermittent ultrasound imaging is recommended to ensure that the patient remains free of complications while awaiting stone passage.

Beyond Stone Passage

In its most classic form, nephrolithiasis manifests as renal colic. After an acute episode of renal colic is over if the stone is retrieved, it should be sent for analysis. Patient should undergo an evaluation for possible underlying risk factors of nephrolithiasis. These evaluations can help direct the clinician to the specific treatments. Patients with metabolically active stones, children, all non-calcium stone formers, and those patients in demographic groups not typically susceptible to stone formation merit an extensive metabolic evaluation.

While it is uniformly recognized that patients with multiple stones deserve a detailed investigation into the cause of their nephrolithiasis, the evaluation of the patient with a single stone has been the subject of much debate. At this time, the consensus is that all patients, even those with a single stone, should undergo at least a basic evaluation to rule out a systemic etiologic mechanism. [89]

Current medical treatment will not dissolve most stones. It is directed to inhibit stone growth and to prevent the formation of new stones. Medical treatment can be divided into specific therapies based upon the biochemical abnormalities and type of stone present and general nonspecific therapies applicable to all types of stones.

Nonspecific Therapy

Nonspecific therapy primarily consists of increased fluid intake and dietary recommendations as previously discussed.

Specific Therapy According to Stone Composition

Calcium Stone

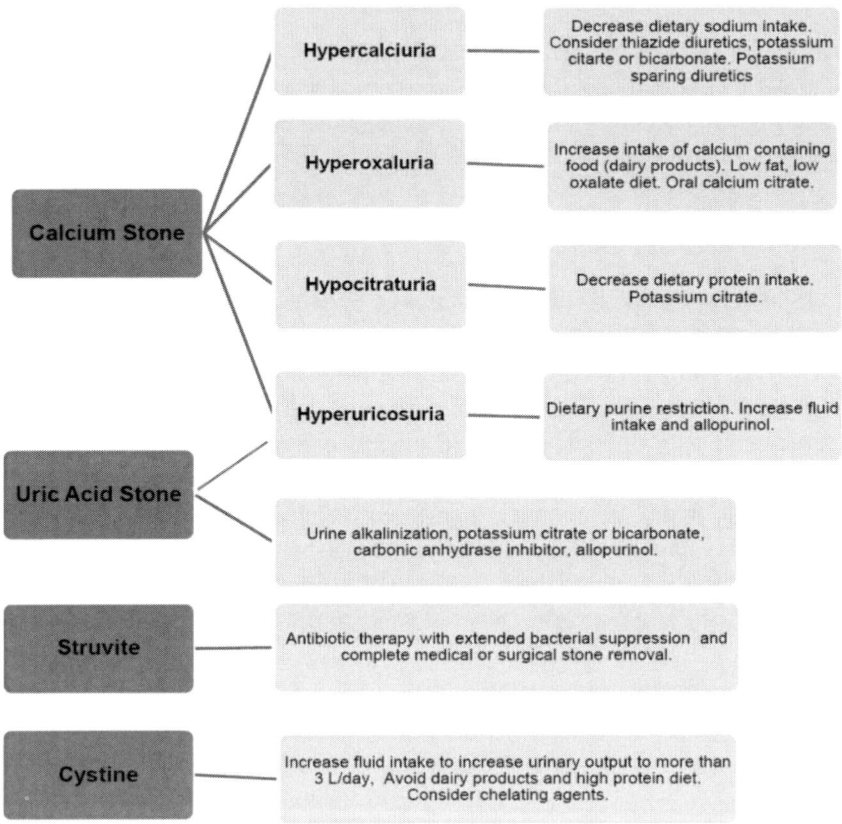

Figure 3. Specific medical preventive therapy for recurrent kidney stones.

Patients who continue to form stones despite dietary modifications often benefit from pharmacologic intervention. Contrary to previously held beliefs, it has become evident that most patients with nephrolithiasis have more than one abnormality of urinary metabolite excretion. Of these, hypercalciuria is the most common abnormality present. Patients with hypercalciuria benefit from thiazides diuretics. Thiazides are an inexpensive and effective means of reducing urinary calcium excretion. To maximize the efficacy of thiazides patients should follow a low sodium diet.

Among thiazide diuretics, chlorthalidone is preferred over hydrochlorothiazide because of its longer half-life. The standard starting dose of chlorthalidone is 25 mg daily. If necessary, this can be uptitrated to 50 mg daily. In patients with dyslipidemia, other cardiovascular risk factors, or elevated blood glucose levels, use of indapamide should be considered as an alternative to thiazides as it has less adverse effects on lipids and blood glucose levels when compared to thiazide medications. [90]

As thiazides can decrease serum potassium levels, patients treated with these medications should be encouraged to increase their dietary intake of foods rich in potassium such as fruits and vegetables. If increased dietary intake of potassium proves inadequate potassium preparations for supplementation such as potassium bicarbonate or citrate can be use. Potassium citrate is the preferred option due to its additional effect of increasing urinary pH. However, it can be switched to potassium chloride should metabolic alkalosis develop. If potassium supplements prove insufficient in raising potassium levels, potassium sparing diuretics can be added to the patient's treatment regimen. Triamterene should be avoided because it is known to increase the risk of stone formation.

In those patients with hyperuricosuria, therapy typically consists of dietary restriction of purine rich foods and increased intake of fluids. Some treatment plans include the initiation of allopurinol 100 to 300 mg daily. Patients with demonstrated hypocitraturia should be advised to reduce protein intake and be started on potassium citrate. This is the preferred salt because sodium citrate in well known for increasing calcium excretion. In patients with chronic kidney disease potassium and bicarbonate levels should be close monitored to avoid metabolic alkalosis and hyperkalemia and their consequent side effect.

Hyperoxaluria can result from a diet rich in oxalate or from increased oxalate absorption via the gastrointestinal tract. Management of hyperoxaluria involves implementing strategies to diminish intestinal oxalate absorption. [5] Patients are instructed to ingest calcium-containing foods, such as milk. The calcium in milk binds the dietary oxalate and may prevent its absorption. Oral calcium citrate or calcium carbonate supplements (1-4 g/day), taken with meals can also be used to block the absorption of oxalate. Although some of the calcium is absorbed, there is a proportionately greater fall in oxalate excretion.

A low fat, low oxalate diet is another means to decrease oxalate absorption through a reduction of fatty acids and oxalate in the colon. Patients should be provided with a list of high oxalate food to be avoided. Patients with malabsorption and short bowel syndrome should be evaluated carefully when dietary restrictions are recommended. Cholestyramine, which binds both bile acids and oxalate in the intestinal lumen is another treatment option. Oxalobacter forminer can be used to reduce oxalate absorption and urinary oxalate excretion. A gluten-free diet can significantly reduce the hyperoxaluria associated with celiac sprue. Magnesium is an additional inhibitor of stone formation. It can be taken as magnesium oxide at 400 mg by mouth twice a day or as magnesium gluconate at 0.5 to 1 g by mouth three times a day.

Uric Acid Stone

Uric acid stones tend to be round, smooth and yellowish-orange. The three corner stones in the management of uric acid nephrolithiasis are: alkalinization of the urine, increased fluid intake and reduction of uric acid production via reduction in purine intake and use of xanthine oxidase inhibitors. Formation of uric acid stones is associated with a low urinary pH. Ideally, to treat uric acid stones urinary pH should be increased to approximately 6.5-7.0; levels at which existing crystals and stones tend to dissolve. A urinary pH above 7 has been associated with calcium phosphate deposition. Either potassium bicarbonate or potassium citrate can be utilized to alkalinize the urine, with a typical dose between 40 to 80 meq/day. [91] If the urinary pH cannot be raised adequately with potassium supplements, the carbonic anhydrase inhibitor acetazolamide can be used. Nitrazine paper should be prescribed to allow patients to monitor their urinary pH at various times of day and to avoid increasing the urinary pH above 7. Regardless of dietary intervention, hyperuricemia often persist particularly in patients with disorders of cellular metabolism. In these patients, allopurinol can be prescribed at a starting dose of 100 mg/day, increasing to 300 mg/day as needed. [92]

Struvite Stones

Struvite stones are generally formed by bacterial production of urease. Eradication of these stones requires early and aggressive medical and urologic management. Essential features of the management of struvite stones involve complete surgical or medical stone removal, appropriate antibiotic therapy and long term bacterial suppression. These stones can rapidly grow to form large staghorn calculi over a period of weeks to months. Preventing the formation of staghorn calculi is critical as these stones can involve the calyces or entire renal pelvis, and their formation can consequently lead to deterioration of kidney function or even end stage renal disease. [93] Moreover, the risk of sepsis with these stones is also high due to stone infection. As a result, most patients with struvite stones require definitive surgical treatment. Shock-wave lithotripsy (SWL) is often adequate for fragmentation of stones smaller than 2 cm, but percutaneous nephrostolithotomy or a combination of the two procedures is usually required for larger stones. Antibiotic therapy should be implemented based on results of either stone fragment or urine culture. Suppressive antibiotics should continue until cultures remain sterile for three consecutive months. Antibiotics may be discontinued once surveillance urine culture obtained monthly for 1 year remain negative. [94]

Treatment of struvite stones may involve urease inhibition and chemolysis. Chemolysis involves irrigation of the kidney with an acidic solution through a nephrostomy tube or ureteral catheter (rarely used nowadays with the advent of less invasive surgical techniques). Urease inhibition has been proved to reduce stone growth and to prevent new stone formation, but has no impact on bacterial growth or the eradication of previously formed stones. It is considered a palliative care strategy for patients who cannot undergo definitive surgical management. Acetohydroxamic acidis (AHA) is the most common used agent in chemolysis. Patients treated with AHA can experience significant side effects such as palpitations, edema, nausea, vomiting, diarrhea, neurologic symptoms, loss of taste, hallucinations, hair loss, rash, abdominal discomfort, hemolytic anemia, and reticulocytosis. [95] Side effects generally resolve after discontinuation of the medication. The starting dose of acetohydroxamic acid is 250 mg twice a day and if well tolerated can be increased to 250 mg three times daily.

Cystine Stones

The primary goal in patients with cystine stones is to lower the urinary cystine concentration by increasing the cystine solubility. Conservative measures include significantly increasing urinary volume to more than 3 liters/day, alkalinizing the urine with potassium citrate, bicarbonate or acetazolamide, and increasing cystine solubility and excretion. The solubility of cystine can be promoted via thiol containing drugs. Its urinary excretion can be promoted with tiopronin. These agents are always used in conjunction with fluid and alkali therapy. [96]

Chelation therapy with d-penicillamine reduces the concentration of cystine concentration by forming a more soluble compound with cystine. Second-generation and third-generation chelating agents such as α-mercaptoproprionylglycine and bucillamine are available for the same purpose and induce fewer side effects. [97]

Surgical Therapy

The management of acute episodes of kidney stone can require surgical management depending on complications at the time of acute presentation or due to the presence of stones that cannot pass spontaneously due to size and or location. Most stones greater than 10 mm and many of those between 5-10 mm in size will require surgical intervention. Current options for therapy of stones that do not pass include shock wave lithotripsy (SWL), ureteroscopic lithotripsy with electrohydraulic or laser probes, percutaneous nephrolithotomy and laparoscopic stone removal. With the development of new technologies, open surgical stone removal is now rarely needed. The specific procedure used varies according to stone location, size, composition, patient factors, and the expertise of the surgeon.

Shock-Wave Lithotripsy (SWL)

This procedure involves focusing sound waves from a machine outside the body onto the kidney stone to fragment it into smaller pieces or "gravel" that can pass spontaneously. SWL is considered the treatment of choice in 75 % of patients. Best results with SWL is seen in patients with stones smaller than 15mm, located in the renal pelvis or upper ureter which are not composed of cystine or calcium oxalate monohydrate. The procedure has potential short term complications, including fever or urinary tract infection. SWL has been contraindicated in patients with coagulopathy and in pregnant women. Because of its noninvasive nature, SWL is very popular in the treatment of ureteral stones with high stone free rates. This technique is widely available and may require general or regional anesthesia. Data suggest that it may be less successful in patients with a higher body mass index, because of a high skin-to-stone distance. [97,98]

Ureteroscopy (URS)

This technique entails the passage of a semi rigid or flexible scope through the bladder and into the ureter. Is considered the procedure of choice for distal ureteral stones and larger proximal stones. It is also considered the best choice in obese patients, in those with complex renal anatomy or in those with high risk of bleeding. Improvements in fiberoptic lens systems have allowed for the creation of smaller ureteroscopes that can navigate the ureter without prior dilation. Endocorporeal lithotripsy can be added to URS to directly fragment visualized stones. This results in high stone-free rates after the procedure. [99] Complications of URS include urinary tract infection, sepsis, ureteral stricture, ureteral injury, and steinstrasse defined as the linear accumulation of small stones blocking a ureter after fragmentation of a larger stone.

Percutaneous Nephrolithotomy (PNL)

This procedure involves the placement of a large needle through the flank into the renal collecting system. The tract is dilated, and instruments are used to rupture and remove the stone. It is a more invasive procedure but the most effective for removing large (usually >2 cm) stones or staghorn stones. It is the preferred option in infected struvite stones where complete removal of the stone leads to the best outcomes. [100] This technique has been greatly improved since 1980s, due to development of flexible and rigid nephroscopes, and laser or pneumatic lithotripsy via the nephroscope.

Adjunctive Procedures

Nephrostomy tubes are routinely placed in patients undergoing PNL and are also frequently used for drainage of infected stone fragments or pain relief following SWL. Ureteral stents are routinely inserted prior to SWL of staghorn calculi. In many cases, a double-pigtail stent is placed and left indwelling for days or weeks to maintain drainage while fragments pass.

Conclusion

Given the high prevalence of kidney stones and the morbidity associated with this disorder, nephrolithiasis remains a major public health burden. The underlying mechanism of stone formation is complex involving the interplay of multiple organ systems, including the gut, liver, bone and kidney. As a result, the approach to diagnosis and management of nephrolithiasis is multifaceted. Presently, key elements of management include risk factor modification (with particular attention paid to dietary counseling), medical expulsive therapy and surgery. Since there is much to be learned regarding precipitants of renal stone formation, there is a need for ongoing research endeavor in this field.

References

[1] Stamatelou KK, Francis ME, Jones CA, Nyberg LM, Curhan GC. Time trends in reported prevalence of kidney stones in the United States: 1976-1994. *Kidney international* 2003;63:1817-23.

[2] Scales CD, Jr., Smith AC, Hanley JM, Saigal CS, Urologic Diseases in America P. Prevalence of kidney stones in the United States. *European urology* 2012;62:160-5.

[3] Romero V, Akpinar H, Assimos DG. Kidney stones: a global picture of prevalence, incidence, and associated risk factors. *Reviews in urology* 2010;12:e86-96.

[4] Taylor EN, Stampfer MJ, Curhan GC. Obesity, weight gain, and the risk of kidney stones. *JAMA* 2005;293:455-62.

[5] Coe FL, Parks JH, Asplin JR. The pathogenesis and treatment of kidney stones. *The New England journal of medicine* 1992;327:1141-52.

[6] Curhan GC, Taylor EN. 24-h uric acid excretion and the risk of kidney stones. *Kidney international* 2008;73:489-96.

[7] Sorensen MD, Eisner BH, Stone KL, et al. Impact of calcium intake and intestinal calcium absorption on kidney stones in older women: the study of osteoporotic fractures. *The Journal of urology* 2012;187:1287-92.

[8] Frick KK, Bushinsky DA. Molecular mechanisms of primary hypercalciuria. *Journal of the American Society of Nephrology: JASN* 2003;14:1082-95.

[9] Bataille P, Achard JM, Fournier A, et al. Diet, vitamin D and vertebral mineral density in hypercalciuric calcium stone formers. *Kidney international* 1991;39:1193-205.

[10] Gambaro G, Vezzoli G, Casari G, Rampoldi L, D'Angelo A, Borghi L. Genetics of hypercalciuria and calcium nephrolithiasis: from the rare monogenic to the common polygenic forms. *American journal of kidney diseases: the official journal of the National Kidney Foundation* 2004;44:963-86.

[11] Lemann J, Jr., Worcester EM, Gray RW. Hypercalciuria and stones. American journal of kidney diseases: the official journal of the National Kidney Foundation 1991;17:386-91.

[12] Moe OW, Bonny O. Genetic hypercalciuria. *Journal of the American Society of Nephrology: JASN* 2005;16:729-45.

[13] Reed BY, Heller HJ, Gitomer WL, Pak CY. Mapping a gene defect in absorptive hypercalciuria to chromosome 1q23.3-q24. *The Journal of clinical endocrinology and metabolism* 1999;84:3907-13.

[14] Wolf MT, Zalewski I, Martin FC, et al. Mapping a new suggestive gene locus for autosomal dominant nephrolithiasis to chromosome 9q33.2-q34.2 by total genome search for linkage. *Nephrology, dialysis, transplantation: official publication of the European Dialysis and Transplant Association - European Renal Association* 2005;20:909-14.

[15] Holmes RP, Goodman HO, Assimos DG. Contribution of dietary oxalate to urinary oxalate excretion. *Kidney international* 2001;59:270-6.

[16] Taylor EN, Curhan GC. Differences in 24-hour urine composition between black and white women. *Journal of the American Society of Nephrology: JASN* 2007;18:654-9.

[17] Smith LH. Diet and hyperoxaluria in the syndrome of idiopathic calcium oxalate urolithiasis. *American journal of kidney diseases: the official journal of the National Kidney Foundation* 1991;17:370-5.

[18] Obialo CI, Clayman RV, Matts JP, et al. Pathogenesis of nephrolithiasis post-partial ileal bypass surgery: case-control study. The POSCH Group. *Kidney international* 1991;39:1249-54.

[19] Williams HE. Oxalic acid and the hyperoxaluric syndromes. *Kidney international* 1978;13:410-7.

[20] Duncan SH, Richardson AJ, Kaul P, Holmes RP, Allison MJ, Stewart CS. Oxalobacter formigenes and its potential role in human health. *Applied and environmental microbiology* 2002;68:3841-7.

[21] Hatch M, Cornelius J, Allison M, Sidhu H, Peck A, Freel RW. Oxalobacter sp. reduces urinary oxalate excretion by promoting enteric oxalate secretion. *Kidney international* 2006;69:691-8.

[22] Kaufman DW, Kelly JP, Curhan GC, et al. Oxalobacter formigenes may reduce the risk of calcium oxalate kidney stones. *Journal of the American Society of Nephrology: JASN* 2008;19:1197-203.

[23] Watts RW. Primary hyperoxaluria type I. *QJM: monthly journal of the Association of Physicians* 1994;87:593-600.

[24] Urivetzky M, Kessaris D, Smith AD. Ascorbic acid overdosing: a risk factor for calcium oxalate nephrolithiasis. *The Journal of urology* 1992;147:1215-8.

[25] Millman S, Strauss AL, Parks JH, Coe FL. Pathogenesis and clinical course of mixed calcium oxalate and uric acid nephrolithiasis. *Kidney international* 1982;22:366-70.

[26] Asplin JR, Parks JH, Chen MS, et al. Reduced crystallization inhibition by urine from men with nephrolithiasis. *Kidney international* 1999;56:1505-16.

[27] Parks JH, Coe FL. A urinary calcium-citrate index for the evaluation of nephrolithiasis. *Kidney international* 1986;30:85-90.

[28] Rudman D, Kutner MH, Redd SC, 2nd, Waters WCt, Gerron GG, Bleier J. Hypocitraturia in calcium nephrolithiasis. *The Journal of clinical endocrinology and metabolism* 1982;55:1052-7.

[29] Wesson JA, Johnson RJ, Mazzali M, et al. Osteopontin is a critical inhibitor of calcium oxalate crystal formation and retention in renal tubules. *Journal of the American Society of Nephrology: JASN* 2003;14:139-47.

[30] Sakhaee K, Alpern R, Poindexter J, Pak CY. Citraturic response to oral citric acid load. *The Journal of urology* 1992;147:975-6.

[31] Demigne C, Sabboh H, Puel C, Remesy C, Coxam V. Organic anions and potassium salts in nutrition and metabolism. *Nutrition research reviews* 2004;17:249-58.

[32] Asplin JR, Arsenault D, Parks JH, Coe FL, Hoyer JR. Contribution of human uropontin to inhibition of calcium oxalate crystallization. *Kidney international* 1998;53:194-9.

[33] Hess B, Zipperle L, Jaeger P. Citrate and calcium effects on Tamm-Horsfall glycoprotein as a modifier of calcium oxalate crystal aggregation. *The American journal of physiology* 1993;265:F784-91.

[34] Lieske JC, Toback FG. Regulation of renal epithelial cell endocytosis of calcium oxalate monohydrate crystals. *The American journal of physiology* 1993;264:F800-7.

[35] Monk RD. Clinical approach to adults. *Seminars in nephrology* 1996;16:375-88.

[36] Monk RD, Bushinky DA. Nephrolithiasis and Nephrocalcinosis. In: Frehally J, Floege J, Johnson RJ, eds. *Comprehensive Clinical Nephrology. London, UK: Mosby;* 2007:641-55.

[37] Taylor EN, Stampfer MJ, Curhan GC. Dietary factors and the risk of incident kidney stones in men: new insights after 14 years of follow-up. *Journal of the American Society of Nephrology: JASN* 2004;15:3225-32.

[38] Curhan GC, Willett WC, Rimm EB, Stampfer MJ. Family history and risk of kidney stones. *Journal of the American Society of Nephrology: JASN* 1997;8:1568 73.

[39] Uribarri J, Oh MS, Carroll HJ. The first kidney stone. *Annals of internal medicine* 1989;111:1006-9.

[40] Carr MC, Prien EL, Jr., Babayan RK. Triamterene nephrolithiasis: renewed attention is warranted. *The Journal of urology* 1990;144:1339-40.

[41] Kopp JB, Miller KD, Mican JA, et al. Crystalluria and urinary tract abnormalities associated with indinavir. *Annals of internal medicine* 1997;127:119-25.

[42] Sasson JP, Dratch PL, Shortsleeve MJ. Renal US findings in sulfadiazine-induced crystalluria. *Radiology* 1992;185:739-40.

[43] Ferraro PM, Taylor EN, Gambaro G, Curhan GC. Soda and other beverages and the risk of kidney stones. *Clinical journal of the American Society of Nephrology: CJASN* 2013;8:1389-95.

[44] Curhan GC, Willett WC, Rimm EB, Speizer FE, Stampfer MJ. Body size and risk of kidney stones. *Journal of the American Society of Nephrology: JASN* 1998;9:1645-52.

[45] Curhan GC, Willett WC, Rimm EB, Spiegelman D, Stampfer MJ. Prospective study of beverage use and the risk of kidney stones. *American journal of epidemiology* 1996;143:240-7.

[46] Bek-Jensen H, Fornander AM, Nilsson MA, Tiselius HG. Is citrate an inhibitor of calcium oxalate crystal growth in high concentrations of urine? *Urological research* 1996;24:67-71.

[47] Honow R, Laube N, Schneider A, Kessler T, Hesse A. Influence of grapefruit-, orange- and apple-juice consumption on urinary variables

and risk of crystallization. *The British journal of nutrition* 2003;90:295-300.

[48] Odvina CV. Comparative value of orange juice versus lemonade in reducing stone-forming risk. *Clinical journal of the American Society of Nephrology: CJASN* 2006;1:1269-74.

[49] Seltzer MA, Low RK, McDonald M, Shami GS, Stoller ML. Dietary manipulation with lemonade to treat hypocitraturic calcium nephrolithiasis. *The Journal of urology* 1996;156:907-9.

[50] Frassetto L, Kohlstadt I. Treatment and prevention of kidney stones: an update. *American family physician* 2011;84:1234-42.

[51] Acar B, Inci Arikan F, Emeksiz S, Dallar Y. Risk factors for nephrolithiasis in children. *World journal of urology* 2008;26:627-30.

[52] Sas DJ, Hulsey TC, Shatat IF, Orak JK. Increasing incidence of kidney stones in children evaluated in the emergency department. *The Journal of pediatrics* 2010;157:132-7.

[53] Ross AE, Handa S, Lingeman JE, Matlaga BR. Kidney stones during pregnancy: an investigation into stone composition. *Urological research* 2008;36:99-102.

[54] Swartz MA, Lydon-Rochelle MT, Simon D, Wright JL, Porter MP. Admission for nephrolithiasis in pregnancy and risk of adverse birth outcomes. *Obstetrics and gynecology* 2007;109:1099-104.

[55] Ogden CL, Carroll MD, Kit BK, Flegal KM. Prevalence of childhood and adult obesity in the United States, 2011-2012. *JAMA* 2014;311:806-14.

[56] Powell CR, Stoller ML, Schwartz BF, et al. Impact of body weight on urinary electrolytes in urinary stone formers. *Urology* 2000;55:825-30.

[57] Nishio S, Yokoyama M, Iwata H, et al. [Obesity as one of the risk factors for urolithiasis]. *Nihon Hinyokika Gakkai zasshi The japanese journal of urology* 1998;89:573-80.

[58] Al-Hayek S, Schwen ZR, Jackman SV, Averch TD. The impact of obesity on urine composition and nephrolithiasis management. *Journal of endourology / Endourological Society* 2013;27:379-83.

[59] Ekeruo WO, Tan YH, Young MD, et al. Metabolic risk factors and the impact of medical therapy on the management of nephrolithiasis in obese patients. *The Journal of urology* 2004;172:159-63.

[60] Ettinger B, Pak CY, Citron JT, Thomas C, Adams-Huet B, Vangessel A. Potassium-magnesium citrate is an effective prophylaxis against recurrent calcium oxalate nephrolithiasis. *The Journal of urology* 1997;158:2069-73.

[61] Borghi L, Meschi T, Amato F, Briganti A, Novarini A, Giannini A. Urinary volume, water and recurrences in idiopathic calcium nephrolithiasis: a 5-year randomized prospective study. *The Journal of urology* 1996;155:839-43.

[62] Gettman MT, Ogan K, Brinkley LJ, Adams-Huet B, Pak CY, Pearle MS. Effect of cranberry juice consumption on urinary stone risk factors. *The Journal of urology* 2005;174:590-4; quiz 801.

[63] Wabner CL, Pak CY. Effect of orange juice consumption on urinary stone risk factors. *The Journal of urology* 1993;149:1405-8.

[64] Fox IH, Kelley WN. Studies on the mechanism of fructose-induced hyperuricemia in man. *Metabolism: clinical and experimental* 1972;21:713-21.

[65] Nguyen NU, Dumoulin G, Henriet MT, Regnard J. Increase in urinary calcium and oxalate after fructose infusion. *Hormone and metabolic research = Hormon- und Stoffwechselforschung = Hormones et metabolisme* 1995;27:155-8.

[66] Taylor EN, Curhan GC. Fructose consumption and the risk of kidney stones. *Kidney international* 2008;73:207-12.

[67] Eisner BH, Asplin JR, Goldfarb DS, Ahmad A, Stoller ML. Citrate, malate and alkali content in commonly consumed diet sodas: implications for nephrolithiasis treatment. *The Journal of urology* 2010;183:2419-23.

[68] Borghi L, Schianchi T, Meschi T, et al. Comparison of two diets for the prevention of recurrent stones in idiopathic hypercalciuria. *The New England journal of medicine* 2002;346:77-84.

[69] Breslau NA, Brinkley L, Hill KD, Pak CY. Relationship of animal protein-rich diet to kidney stone formation and calcium metabolism. *The Journal of clinical endocrinology and metabolism* 1988;66:140-6.

[70] Evan AP, Lingeman JE, Coe FL, et al. Randall's plaque of patients with nephrolithiasis begins in basement membranes of thin loops of Henle. *The Journal of clinical investigation* 2003;111:607-16.

[71] Dussol B, Iovanna C, Rotily M, et al. A randomized trial of low-animal-protein or high-fiber diets for secondary prevention of calcium nephrolithiasis. *Nephron Clinical practice* 2008;110:c185-94.

[72] Kok DJ, Khan SR. Calcium oxalate nephrolithiasis, a free or fixed particle disease. *Kidney international* 1994;46:847-54.

[73] Meschi T, Maggiore U, Fiaccadori E, et al. The effect of fruits and vegetables on urinary stone risk factors. *Kidney international* 2004;66:2402-10.

[74] Curhan GC, Willett WC, Rimm EB, Stampfer MJ. A prospective study of dietary calcium and other nutrients and the risk of symptomatic kidney stones. *The New England journal of medicine* 1993;328:833-8.

[75] Curhan GC, Knight EL, Rosner B, Hankinson SE, Stampfer MJ. Lifetime nonnarcotic analgesic use and decline in renal function in women. *Archives of internal medicine* 2004;164:1519-24.

[76] Lemann J, Jr., Piering WF, Lennon EJ. Possible role of carbohydrate-induced calciuria in calcium oxalate kidney-stone formation. *The New England journal of medicine* 1969;280:232-7.

[77] Curhan GC, Willett WC, Knight EL, Stampfer MJ. Dietary factors and the risk of incident kidney stones in younger women: Nurses' Health Study II. *Archives of internal medicine* 2004;164:885-91.

[78] Asplin JR, Donahue S, Kinder J, Coe FL. Urine calcium excretion predicts bone loss in idiopathic hypercalciuria. *Kidney international* 2006;70:1463-7.

[79] Taylor EN, Curhan GC. Diet and fluid prescription in stone disease. *Kidney international* 2006;70:835-9.

[80] Preminger GM, Tiselius HG, Assimos DG, et al. 2007 guideline for the management of ureteral calculi. *The Journal of urolog*y 2007;178:2418-34.

[81] Cole RS, Fry CH, Shuttleworth KE. The action of the prostaglandins on isolated human ureteric smooth muscle. *British journal of urology* 1988;61:19-26.

[82] Springhart WP, Marguet CG, Sur RL, et al. Forced versus minimal intravenous hydration in the management of acute renal colic: a randomized trial. *Journal of endourology / Endourological Society* 2006;20:713-6.

[83] Holdgate A, Pollock T. Systematic review of the relative efficacy of non-steroidal anti-inflammatory drugs and opioids in the treatment of acute renal colic. *BMJ* 2004;328:1401.

[84] Laird JM, Roza C, Cervero F. Effects of artificial calculosis on rat ureter motility: peripheral contribution to the pain of ureteric colic. *The American journal of physiology* 1997;272:R1409-16.

[85] Sivula A, Lehtonen T. Spontaneous passage of artificial concretions applied in the rabbit ureter. *Scandinavian journal of urology and nephrology* 1967;1:259-63.

[86] Maggi CA, Giuliani S. A pharmacological analysis of calcium channels involved in phasic and tonic responses of the guinea-pig ureter to high potassium. *Journal of autonomic pharmacology* 1995;15:55-64.

[87] Morita T, Wada I, Suzuki T, Tsuchida S. Characterization of alpha-adrenoceptor subtypes involved in regulation of ureteral fluid transport. *The Tohoku journal of experimental medicine* 1987;152:111-8.

[88] Hollingsworth JM, Rogers MA, Kaufman SR, et al. Medical therapy to facilitate urinary stone passage: a meta-analysis. *Lancet* 2006;368:1171-9.

[89] Consensus conference. Prevention and treatment of kidney stones. *JAMA* 1988;260:977-81.

[90] Borghi L, Meschi T, Guerra A, Novarini A. Randomized prospective study of a nonthiazide diuretic, indapamide, in preventing calcium stone recurrences. *Journal of cardiovascular pharmacology* 1993;22 Suppl 6:S78-86.

[91] Kenny JE, Goldfarb DS. Update on the pathophysiology and management of uric acid renal stones. *Current rheumatology reports* 2010;12:125-9.

[92] Ettinger B, Tang A, Citron JT, Livermore B, Williams T. Randomized trial of allopurinol in the prevention of calcium oxalate calculi. The New England journal of medicine 1986;315:1386-9.

[93] Jungers P, Joly D, Barbey F, Choukroun G, Daudon M. ESRD caused by nephrolithiasis: prevalence, mechanisms, and prevention. *American journal of kidney diseases: the official journal of the National Kidney Foundation* 2004;44:799-805.

[94] Preminger GM, Assimos DG, Lingeman JE, et al. Chapter 1: AUA guideline on management of staghorn calculi: diagnosis and treatment recommendations. *The Journal of urology* 2005;173:1991-2000.

[95] Wong HY, Reidl CR, Griffith DP. Medical management and prevention of struvite stones. In: Coe FL, Favus MJ, Pak CYC, eds. Kidney stones; Medical and Surgical management. Philadelphia, PA: Lippincott-Raven; 1996:941-50.

[96] Asplin DM, Asplin JR. The Interaction of thiol drugs and urine pH in the treatment of cystinuria. *The Journal of urology* 2013;189:2147-51.

[97] Sakhaee K. Pathogenesis and medical management of cystinuria. *Seminars in nephrology* 1996;16:435-47.

[98] Putman SS, Hamilton BD, Johnson DB. The use of shock wave lithotripsy for renal calculi. *Current opinion in urology* 2004;14:117-21.

[99] Leveillee RJ, Lobik L. Intracorporeal lithotripsy: which modality is best? *Current opinion in urology* 2003;13:249-53.

[100] Samplaski MK, Irwin BH, Desai M. Less-invasive ways to remove stones from the kidneys and ureters. *Cleveland Clinic journal of medicine* 2009;76:592-8.

In: Nephrolithiasis
Editor: Melody Shneider
ISBN: 978-1-63482-134-6

Chapter II

Uric Acid Nephrolithiasis

***Milagros Zegarra*[1], *Rupam Ruchi*[2,*], *Kimberly Hammer*[1] *and Tze Shien Lo*[1]**
[1]VAMC-Fargo Virginia, US
[2]University of Florida, Gainesville, Florida, US

Abstract

Uric acid nephrolithiasis accounts for 5–10 % of all kidney stones in the general population in the United States (US) and is noted to be increasing in other parts of the world like Japan, previously known to have a low incidence of this condition. This increase is attributable, at least in part, to westernized eating habits.

The prevalence of uric acid nephrolithiasis has continued to rise at alarming rates in high risk populations, such as patients with type 2 diabetes mellitus, obesity and metabolic syndrome. In these conditions, there are changes in the serum and urine chemistries leading to more acidic urine and chronically increased uric acid production, which are both pre-requisites for the formation of uric acid stones.

The clinical presentation is similar to any other kidney stone that includes pain radiating from the flank into the pelvic area, as the stone moves downward, and concomitant associated symptoms such as nausea, vomiting, fever and hematuria can be also present. These stones are

* Corresponding author: Rupam Ruchi, email: rupadoc@gmail.com.

diagnosed by CT as plain x-rays are not helpful since uric acid stones are not radiopaque. The treatment for uric acid stones is well-defined nowadays; consisting of alkalinizing the urine and increasing fluid intake, and in selected cases, the use of xanthine oxidase inhibitors might be needed.

In this review, we focus on the pathophysiology diagnoses, causes, treatment and prevention of uric acid stones.

Epidemiology

The occurrence of nephrolithiasis has been increasing globally. The prevalence of kidney stones in United States has doubled from 2.6% in 1960s to 5.2% in 1990s [1]. 12% men and 6% women will develop a kidney stone in their lifetime. In 2012, a study by National Health and Nutrition Examination Survey (NHANES) found the prevalence to be 8.8%, an increase from 5.2% it found in 1994 [2,3]. Similar increase has been reported from European and Asian countries, including Germany, Spain, Japan and Korea [4,5].

Uric acid stones are the second most common type after calcium oxalate, comprising 5-10% of all renal stones [6]. An analysis of VA population for renal calculi revealed that 10% of patients had at least some component of uric acid in their stones, while 9.7% had pure uric acid stones [7]. As with other stones, the incidence of uric acid stones has also increased from 5.6% to 8.1% over 3 decades [8]. Geographic variation is known to occur, with uric acid stone rates varying between 4-40% [9], suggesting the role of genetic and environmental factors in etiology. Furthermore, uric acid or sodium urate precipitation provides a nidus for subsequent formation of calcium oxalate stones (mixed uric acid-calcium oxalate stones), thus the actual incidence may be higher. Calcium oxalate stones can also occur from uric acid induced crystallization of calcium salts (mixed stones) [10].

Uric Acid Metabolism

Uric acid is the end product of purine metabolism. Endogenous as well as dietary purines are metabolized to hypoxanthine and xanthine, which are then converted to uric acid by an enzyme called xanthine oxidase. Uric acid is poorly soluble; hence some mammals have another enzyme called uric acid oxidase, to catalyze the breakdown of uric acid into allantoin, a more soluble substance than uric acid itself. However, humans have lost this enzyme to evolution [11]. Thus the level of uric acid in humans is significantly higher than in certain other mammals (Figure 1).

Uric acid is a weak acid, and exists in equilibrium with its base urate. The pKa of this reaction is 5.35 at body temperature. At pH of 7.40, the direction of this reaction is to the right; implying most of the uric acid exists in blood in the form of its conjugate base (urate). In the urine, at a pH of 5.5 for example, the direction of the reaction remains to the right, but less so in terms of magnitude. However, as urine becomes more acidic, the direction of the reaction shifts to the left, leading to higher concentration of undissociated uric acid (Figure 1).

Table 1. Etiology and risk factors for uric acid stones. In most patients, it is a combination of these factors that predispose them to uric acid stones

1. Low urine pH
• Insulin resistance (Metabolic syndrome*)
• Chronic diarrhea**
• Renal acidification defect (Renal tubular acidosis)
• High dietary acid load (high protein/low carbohydrate diet, alcohol)
2. Hyperuricosuria
• High serum uric acid
a. Idiopathic hyperuricemic gout (metabolic syndrome*)
b. Myeloproliferative syndrome, other malignancies with high tumor burden
c. Congenital enzyme deficiencies of uric acid metabolism
d. Psoriasis
• Low to normal serum uric acid
a. Drugs: Probenecid, Losartan, High dose salicylates
b. Familial hypouricemic hyperuricosuria
3. Low urine volume
• Chronic diarrhea**
• High output ileostomies
• Acute gastroenteritis
• Reduced fluid intake
• Volume loss due to excessive sweatin

*Predispose to stones by being associated with high serum uric acid and acidic urine. Comprises of a combination of obesity, impaired glucose tolerance, hypertension, dyslipidemia

**Predispose to stones by causing acidic urine and low urine volume

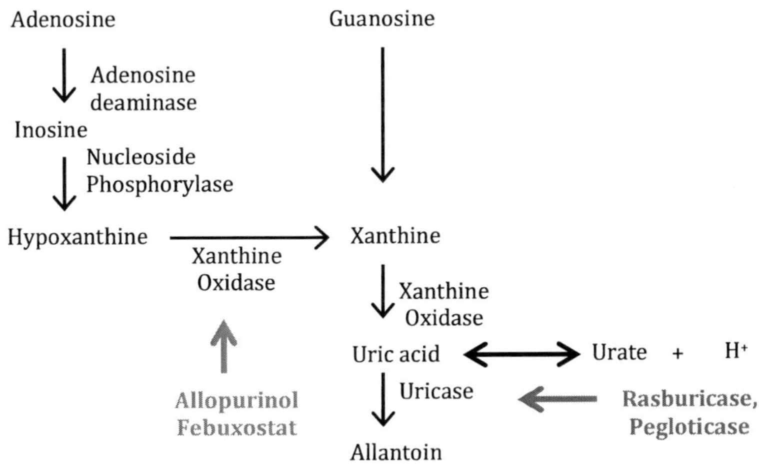

Figure 1. depicting normal purine metabolism and uric acid pathway. Uricase enzyme is not present in humans, however recombinant enzyme such as Rasburicase and Pegylated form of the enzyme, Pegloticase are used to treat hyperuricemia. Allopurinol is a structural analog of hypoxanthine and thus a non-specific xanthine oxidase inhibitor, whereas febuxostat is a synthetic, specific inhibitor of the enzyme. Uric acid is a weak acid that exists in equilibrium with its conjugate base (Urate$^-$) and H^+, at a pH of 5.35. In solutions with higher pH like blood, urate is predominant, whereas in solutions with lower pH like acidic urine, uric acid is the predominant form.

Risk Factors and Etiology

The solubility of uric acid in a solution is 96 mg/L. Precipitation occurs whenever the solubility threshold is exceeded. While low urine volume and high uric acid excretion can increase the concentration of uric acid in the urine, the role of urine pH remains paramount. Accordingly, the conditions associated with increased risk of uric acid stone formation can be broadly categorized as shown in table 1, and elaborated below:

1. Conditions Associated with Low Urine pH, Typically below 5.5

As discussed above, the concentration of undissociated uric acid in the urine not only depends upon total amount of uric acid, but also on the urine pH. As an estimate, at a pH of 5.35, approximately 200 mg/L of uric acid can be present before it exceeds its solubility. By contrast, at a pH of 6.5, up to

1200 mg/L of total uric acid may be present without exceeding its solubility [6]. Patients who form uric acid stones typically have a lower urine pH than others. A study comparing 56 patients who had idiopathic uric acid stones with 54 patients who had calcium oxalate stones, found that the former group had a significantly lower mean urinary pH than the latter (5.34 versus 6.17), primarily due to impaired ammoniagenesis [12,13].

Patients with high dietary acid load (for example, excessive consumption of low carbohydrate high protein diet [14]), chronic diarrhea, renal acidification defects (renal tubular acidosis) have low urine pH, and are hence predisposed to uric acid stones. More commonly however, uric acid stones are seen in people with none of these risk factors. Rather, such patients usually have idiopathic or primary gout characterized by high serum uric acid, and associated with key features of metabolic syndrome like hypertension, obesity, impaired glucose tolerance and dyslipidemia [15]. Diabetes in particular, has recently emerged as an independent strong factor for development of uric acid stones. Among diabetics, uric acid stones constitute approximately 34% of all stones [16]. In one study, the proportion of patients with type II diabetes in uric acid stone formers was 27.8% as compared to 6.8% in calcium stone formers [17]. Obesity itself is a strong risk factor for uric acid stone formation, accounting for up to 63% of all stones in this cohort [18,19]. Both obesity and diabetes are integral part of metabolic syndrome, which is also associated with dyslipidemia and hypertension, and is characterized by insulin resistance. Hypertriglyceridemia itself has been shown to be associated with uric acid stone formation [13].

There is now ample evidence to suggest a strong association between metabolic syndrome and uric acid nephrolithiasis. In fact, rising incidence of metabolic syndrome is epidemiologically consistent with the rise in incidence of uric acid stones. Interestingly, the odds of getting uric acid stone are proportionate to the number of traits of metabolic syndrome a patient has. For example, the odds ratio increases from 1.1 in patients with a single trait, to 1.8 in those with four. Another study reported an increase in proportion of uric acid stones from 10.2% in those with one trait to 30.4% in those with four [20,21]. It is to be noted though that both studies were done in Japanese population. The key factor linking metabolic syndrome with uric acid nephrolithiasis is low urine pH. Insulin promotes ammoniagenesis by several mechanisms. It stimulates phosphate dependent glutaminase, an enzyme that catalyzes the formation of glutamate and ammonium from glutamine in renal proximal tubular cells [22]. Insulin also stimulates the sodium-hydrogen exchanger (NHE-3) in these cells, thus overall stimulatinges ammoniagenesis

[23]. Insulin resistance is therefore a state of reduced ammoniagenesis, thereby limiting the ability of the kidneys to buffer hydrogen ions. Additionally, glutamine metabolism provides substrate (such as alpha ketoglutarate) for citric acid cycle, thus serving as a source of ATP. In the presence of insulin resistance however, there is excess of free fatty acids in circulation, which serve as alternate source of energy, thus decreasing the dependence of kidneys on glutamine. Reduced glutamine metabolism in turn results in decreased ammoniagenesis.

Indeed in a controlled study, Sakhee et al. showed that urine pH was significantly low in patients with uric acid nephrolithiasis and insulin resistance. But even in subjects without uric acid stones, Abate et al. showed that those with insulin resistance had lower urinary pH. When they compared the stone formers from non-stone formers on a controlled diet, those with uric acid stones had lower pH. The fraction of net acid excreted as ammonium was found to be lower in these patients, but the net acid excretion was maintained by higher titratable acid and lower citrate [24].

2. Conditions Associated with High Uric Acid Excretion

Hyperuricosuria can be associated with high serum uric acid (hyperuricemic hyperuricosuria) or normal/low uric acid levels (normal/hypouricemic hyperuricosuria). Former category includes conditions with high cell turnover, like myeloproliferative syndrome, other malignancies with high tumor burden, use of chemotherapeutic agents, psoriasis, congenital syndromes of purine metabolism, such as hypoxanthine-guanine phosphoribosyl transferase (HPRT) deficiency, PRPP (phosphoribosyl pyrophosphate) synthetase overactivity, glucose-6 phosphate dehydrogenase deficiency (Von Gierke disease), glycogen storage disorders (type III, V and VII). All these enzyme abnormalities lead to increased purine production or excessive breakdown of intermediary molecules in nucleotide metabolism, leading to increased uric acid accumulation [25]. Primary gout is another condition in which hyperuricemia can lead to increased uric acid excretion and crystallization in presence of low urinary pH. Indeed 10-20% of patients with primary gout and normouricosuria develop uric acid stones, once again underlying the importance of urine pH in stone formation. In patients with primary gout and hyperuricosuria, this incidence can be as high as 40% [26].

On the other hand, certain uricosuric drugs like probenecid, losartan and high dose salicylates act on the renal tubules to increase uric acid excretion.

Since production is not affected, the serum levels of uric acid remain in the low to low-normal range. Losartan and probenecid are potent inhibitors of uric acid reabsorption through urate-anion exchange transporter [27], specifically URAT1 located on the luminal side of proximal tubular cells [28]. This effect of losartan is independent of its inhibitory effect on renin-angiotensin system.

Of note, loop diuretics and thiazide diuretics cause hyperuricemia directly by inhibiting urate secretion in the proximal tubules, as well as indirectly by causing decreased filtration and increased reabsorption via effects of volume depletion [29]. However, since the cause of hyperuricemia is decreased renal clearance, they typically do not cause hyperuricosuria and stones.

3. Conditions Associated with Low Urine Volume

Volume depletion caused by diarrhea, vomiting, excessive sweating, inadequate oral intake can cause low urine volume, thereby predisposing to uric acid precipitation. By itself, it is insufficient to cause uric acid stones. However, it creates an environment conducive to stone formation, in predisposed individuals.

Pathogenesis

All uric acid stones have an organic matrix and an inorganic component made of uric acid crystals. The matrix comprises 2-3% of the weight of these stones and majority of it is protein. Both the organic and inorganic components of the stone are arranged in parallel concentric laminations. The matrix deposition precedes the crystal formation, and is thought to play an important role in regulating crystallization [30,31]. In a study on proteomic analysis of uric acid stone matrix, authors found that most proteins were involved in the inflammation pathway via complement system, phagocytosis or IL-6 [30]. This suggests the role of inflammation in stone formation. Similar studies on calcium oxalate stones have also suggested the role of inflammation and cell injury in stone formation [32]. Presence of stone inhibitors and promoters has been well studied for calcium oxalate stones, however data for such proteins/compounds for uric acid stones is limited.

The first step in crystallization is nucleation on a foreign surface (heterogeneous nucleation). Homogenous nucleation is a possibility but requires a very high level of supersaturation, unlike the heterogeneous process where the foreign surface acts as a catalyst of nucleation. High or low, a supersaturation barrier must still be overcome for nucleation to occur. Thereafter, a stone may increase in size simply by direct incorporation of crystal onto the lattice (also known as growth) and by another process called aggregation. In the urine, crystals randomly collide with each other, and while some disperse, others may aggregate together. The net effect is determined by an efficiency factor, and if aggregation is predominant, then consolidation of several crystals can occur to cause increase in crystal mass [33]. Uric acid crystallizes either in the form of monoclinic anhydrous uric acid or in the rhomboid dihydrous form of uric acid. While both forms commonly occur together in most stones, the transformation of one into another is dependent on temperature, pH and solute concentration [34].

Clinical Features

Signs and Symptoms

Uric acid nephrolithiasis can present with a wide range of clinical features from an asymptomatic incidental finding to a passage of gravel material or acute obstruction.

Symptoms usually develop when the stone moves from the renal pelvis down to the ureter, this typically manifests as unilateral abdominal pain. The nature of the pain is acute and can vary from mild to severe, lasting for minutes or even days. The pain is paroxysmal as the stone finds it way downwards into the ureter, the intermittent pain is thought to be related to the stretching of the ureters or the renal capsule. The resolution of the pain occurs with passage of the stone or after surgical intervention is performed.

Gross hematuria is a prominent and a common feature related to the trauma produced to the uroepithelium by the stone, but microscopic hematuria by dipstick has also been described.

The interval between the onset of pain and the urine collection has a significant impact on the diagnostic performance of the dipstick test. However negative microscopic hematuria has been described if the test is performed 3 days after the onset of symptoms [35].

Anuria is not a common clinical feature but in certain circumstances complete outlet obstruction can occur, such as in patients with a single working kidney or in transplant recipients.

The location of the pain depends on where the stone is located, if the obstruction occurs in the upper region or near the renal pelvis the patient will present with flank pain, if the stone is lodged in the lower ureteral area the pain will be on the lower quadrant, radiating to the ipsilateral groin, this has classically been known as renal colic.

Stones that are located in the bladder can lead to urinary difficulties such as increase in frequency, nocturia, incontinence and decreased strength; these symptoms result from the inability of the bladder to empty completely.

The physical exam is for the most part unremarkable in adults, besides the reported pain, hypertension or hypotension can be associated and flank tenderness can be triggered in certain circumstances but only rarely can hydronephrosis be palpated in an adult.

Complications

Obstruction will ensue if the stone is unable to pass, if this is left untreated long-term renal damage or even complete renal loss will occur.

As the urine flow is affected, urinary tract infections can present and range from cystitis to pyelonephritis with associated systemic symptoms.

Diagnoses

Once urinary tract obstruction by a stone is suspected, a prompt diagnoses is essential, as timely intervention is directly related to renal recovery

A variety of radiologic techniques have been described, there are two imaging modalities currently recommended, non contrast abdominal computed tomography (NCCT) and ultrasound, NCCT is more sensitive than ultrasonography, while ultrasonography is not associated with radiation.

There has been a lack of consensus about the initial imaging method for patients with suspected nephrolithiasis, and the fact that CT entails exposure to ionizing radiation led to a recent comparison study. *R. Smith-Bindman*, et al. randomized 2759 patients presenting to the emergency department (ED) to point-of-care ultrasonography performed by emergency physicians who had training as recommended by the American College of Emergency Physicians, radiology ultrasonography, and NCCT. The results concluded that ultrasonography was associated with lower cumulative radiation exposure than NCCT, without significant differences in high-risk diagnoses with complications, serious adverse events, pain scores, return visits to the ED nor hospitalizations. Of note is the specificity of NCCT reported in this trial was only 58 percent, lower than the ones reported in other trials, this is likely related to the requirement of visual confirmation of the stone as the diagnostic gold standard[36].

Non-contrast CT (NCCT)

NCCT has a reported median sensitivity and specificity for the detection of ureteral calculi as 98% and 97%, respectively, superior to other imaging modalities. It can also detect signs of urinary tract obstruction, depending on the duration of the acute process [37].

One main issue is that patients with suspected nephrolithiasis will often required repeated imaging studies, so efforts to reduce radiation dose are needed, in certain circumstance low-dose NCCT imaging can be performed, this scan allows for identification of the stone with similar sensitivity and specificity as a standard NCCT scan.

However this technique is not recommended for patients with Body Mass Index (BMI) greater than 30 kg/m2 as the sensitivity and specificity for detecting ureteral stones is lower when compared to conventional NCCT [38]. This technique is also reported to have no statistically significant difference in sensitivity for the detection of calculi greater than 3 mm in diameter [39].

A limitation of NCCT is its use in pregnant patients and either protocol should be avoided.

Ultrasound

Renal colic is the most frequent non-obstetric cause of abdominal pain during pregnancy [40], in this setting renal ultrasonography is used as the first-line diagnostic test because of the availability and lack of ionizing radiation. The disadvantages of this technique are that it is operator dependent, and a lower sensitivity to detect nephrolithiasis during pregnancy ranging from 34 to 92.5 % [41].

It may also be unable to differentiate between ureteral obstruction related to ureterolithiasis and the physiological hydronephrosis related to the mechanical compression of the ureter occurring during pregnancy [42].

24-Hour Urine Collection

The 24-hour urine collection can reveal hyperuricosuria, but this is not necessarily present in all cases. If there is normal urinary uric acid excretion, an acidic urine pH is the primary risk factor for stone formation.

This collection should be obtained a few weeks after the acute episode, if there has not been a stone retrieved for chemical analysis.

Most commercial laboratories offer to calculate the urinary supersaturation of uric acid. This is a parameter that can be followed during treatment; it provides an integrated view of the uric acid excretion, urinary volume and urinary pH.

Treatment

Medical management remains the mainstay of treatment of uric acid nephrolithiasis, and surgical treatment is only rarely indicated. The three cornerstones of therapy target the three pathophysiologic mechanisms of uric acid stone formation, namely low urine pH, hyperuricosuria and low urine output.

1. Urine Alkalization

Urine alkalization is the most important therapeutic measure for dissolution of uric acid stones. Urine pH is paramount in determining the concentration of undissociated uric acid. At a pH of 7, almost all of uric acid exists as the sodium salt of its more soluble conjugate base (monosodium urate). However, such high urinary pH can cause precipitation of calcium phosphate and in turn, lead to formation of phosphate stones. Hence, the urinary pH should be maintained between 6-6.5 [43].

Urine alkalization is difficult to achieve in these patients. Pharmacological options for oral alkalization include sodium bicarbonate (tablets or commercial baking soda), potassium citrate or acetazolamide. Intravenous sodium lactate can be used for a quicker response, but only in patients with a normal functioning liver, which can convert lactate to bicarbonate. Sodium bicarbonate tablets are usually given as 650 mg three times a day. It reacts with hydrochloric acid in the stomach to form carbon dioxide, which produces nausea, belching and abdominal discomfort. Some patients may not be able to tolerate these GI side effects. Also, being a sodium salt of bicarbonate, it can cause edema, hypertension and worsening of heart failure. The incidence of these side effects is much lower with potassium citrate, which is now the preferred first line oral agent for urine alkalization. The usual dose is 30-60 meq per day in divided doses. Being a potassium salt, it can cause hyperkalemia in patients with impaired renal function, or in those who are also taking other medications with a propensity to cause hyperkalemia. These medications include but are not limited to ACE-inhibitors, angiotensin receptor blockers or potassium sparing diuretics including aldosterone antagonists. Acetazolamide is indicated if potassium citrate is unable to increase the urinary pH to the desired range. Being a carbonic anhydrase enzyme inhibitor, it causes bicarbonaturia and elevated urinary pH, but at the cost of inducing acidemia and resultant loss of bone minerals and density over long term. It is also associated with calcium phosphate stones presumably due to increased urine pH. Other side effects include blood dyscrasias, neurological disorders and GI disturbances [44].

There is some evidence that lemon and orange juice have some effect on increasing urine pH and citrate excretion [45,46]. Although not sufficient by themselves, they can act as an adjunct to other treatment modalities, especially in patients who are not able to tolerate high dose of pharmacotherapy.

Oral alkalization of urine is usually effective in causing 80% uric acid stones to dissolve [9]. The time taken for the same usually depends upon the pH and size of the stone. A 2 cm sized pure uric acid stone will take approximately 9 days to dissolve completely at a pH of 7.0 [43]. Percutaneous dissolution of stones using instillation of basic solutions such as sodium bicarbonate or THAM (Tris hydroxymethyl aminomethane, pH 8.6) following percutaneous nephrostomy was often done in the past in patients who did not tolerate or did not respond to oral alkalization. [47,48] However, state of the art endourological techniques available today have obviated the need for such procedures.

2. Targeting Hyperuricosuria

Non-essential drugs causing hyperuricosuria should be discontinued. Efforts should be made to substitute alternative drugs for others. Purine rich dietary products such as red meat, fish and poultry should be avoided. Alcohol can also cause hyperuricemia and should be avoided.

Conditions associated with hyperuricemia should be treated with urate lowering drugs. Depending on their mechanism of action, they can be classified as:

a. Xanthine oxidase inhibitors: Includes drugs such as allopurinol and febuxostat. Both act by inhibiting xanthine oxidase enzyme, thereby reducing the production of uric acid. However they differ in their mechanism of action and side effect profile. Being a structural analog of hypoxanthine, allopurinol competes for the enzyme xanthine oxidase. In the process, it gets converted to oxypurinol, which further binds the enzyme and causes its suicide inhibition. However, this structural similarity also makes it a substrate for other enzymes that eventually affect the pyrimidine synthesis, and are believed to be the cause of several of its side effects including hypersensitive drug reactions [49,50]. Febuxostat, on the other hand, is a synthetic drug, which is a potent but selective inhibitor of xanthine oxidase. Hence, not only it is more effective than allopurinol at decreasing serum uric acid levels, it is also devoid of much of its severe hypersensitivity reactions [51,52]. Both drugs however have the propensity to cause elevated liver enzymes, and musculoskeletal side effects [53]. Allopurinol related severe hypersensitivity syndrome has been reported more commonly in patients with impaired renal function, presumably due to low clearance of oxypurinol, an intermediate active metabolite of allopurinol [54]. In contrast, febuxostat is primarily metabolized in liver, hence is safer in such patients.
b. Recombinant uricase: Include drugs such as rasburicase and pegloticase, which act by breaking down uric acid into the more soluble compound called allantoin. Pegloticase is pegylated form of recombinant uricase, enabling it to be longer-acting than rasburicase. These drugs are only available for parenteral use, and are associated with adverse effects such as infusion reactions, immunogenicity and loss of efficacy upon long term use. These are also expensive, and hence are reserved for acute severe hyperuricemia threatening kidney function, such as that seen post chemotherapy in patients with high tumor burden, or malignancies with rapid turnover such as myeloproliferative disorders.

3. Increasing Urine Volume

Last but not the least, increasing fluid intake to increase the urine volume to 2-2.5 liters a day is helpful to decrease the relative saturation of urine with respect to uric acid, hence preventing its precipitation in urine. It is not specific for uric acid stones, however is an important part of the treatment plan.

Surgical treatment should be considered for those with high-grade obstruction threatening renal function, and presence of infection. It is also indicated in patients not responsive or intolerant to medical therapy. The surgical options are similar as for other stones. ESWL (Extracorporeal shock wave lithotripsy) is a commonly used procedure that breaks down stones into small pieces, which are then flushed out with the urine, or at least become more amenable to medical treatment. Holmium-YAG (laser) lithotripsy is another option. Interestingly, breakage of uric acid stones by Holmium-YAG produces cyanide by a photothermal mechanism, although clinical effects seem insignificant [55].

Prevention

Maintaining alkaline urine, adequate urine output and normal uric acid levels in blood can prevent uric acid stone recurrence. Dietary modification to include more fruits and vegetables, and avoiding excess animal protein helps to maintain a higher urinary pH. Drugs such as potassium citrate, sodium bicarbonate also help. Allopurinol or febuxostat can be used to maintain uric acid in normal range in the blood. Drugs causing hyperuricosuria should be avoided. Patients with myeloproliferative disorders or those on chemotherapy should receive pre-emptive uric acid lowering drugs like allopurinol or febuxostat, before they begin chemotherapy. Uricosuric drugs such as probenecid should be avoided, and urine should be alkalized.

Summary

Incidence of uric acid nephrolithiasis is increasing all over the world, and epidemiologically has paralleled the increase in metabolic syndrome. Low urine pH is the key to uric acid precipitation in the kidney. Hyperuricosuria and low urine volume are other predisposing factors, but by themselves, are unlikely to cause uric acid precipitation unless they are very severe. In most patients, uric acid stones form as a result of an interplay between all these factors. A role of inflammation is also suggested by the presence of inflammation-related proteins in the stone matrix, although the exact mechanism is not clear. Clinical features are similar to any other stone. Diagnostically, uric acid kidney stones are one of the few stones that are radiographically lucent, and hence are not visible on plain X-rays. Non-enhanced CT scan is the diagnostic modality of choice, although the dose of radiation limits its repeated usage over time, as might be needed to follow up for recurrence. In such cases or in acutely symptomatic patients in the emergency room, ultrasound may be the study of choice. Urine analysis for stone parameters other than volume and pH is important for those with mixed uric acid and calcium oxalate stones. Complications include loss of renal function due to prolonged obstruction, and urine infection. Hence, prompt treatment is essential. Treatment is aimed at alkalizing the urine to a goal pH of 6-6.5, lowering the serum uric acid levels and maintaining a urine volume of 2 to 2.5 liters a day. Medical treatment is usually satisfactory, but surgical treatment may be indicated in those with severe obstruction or infection, or in those who do not respond to medical therapy. Prevention of recurrent stones focuses on correcting hyperuricosuria, maintaining an alkaline urine and adequate urine output. Patients with high cell turnover, myeloproliferative syndromes and those on chemotherapy, should receive pre-emptive uric acid lowering drugs along with urine alkalizing therapy.

References

[1] Romero, V; Akpinar, H; Assimos, DG. Kidney stones: a global picture of prevalence, incidence, and associated risk factors. *Reviews in urology*, 2010, 12, e86-96.

[2] Scales, CD, Jr; Smith, AC; Hanley, JM; Saigal, CS. Prevalence of kidney stones in the United States. *European urology*, 2012, 62, 160-5.

[3] Stamatelou, KK; Francis, ME; Jones, CA; Nyberg, LM; Curhan, GC. Time trends in reported prevalence of kidney stones in the United States: 1976-1994. *Kidney international*, 2003, 63, 1817-23.

[4] Hesse, A; Brandle, E; Wilbert, D; Kohrmann, KU; Alken, P. Study on the prevalence and incidence of urolithiasis in Germany comparing the years, 1979 vs., 2000. *European urology*, 2003, 44, 709-13.

[5] Yasui, T; Iguchi, M; Suzuki, S; Kohri, K. Prevalence and epidemiological characteristics of urolithiasis in Japan: national trends between 1965 and, 2005. *Urology*, 2008, 71, 209-13.

[6] Asplin, JR. Uric acid stones. *Seminars in nephrology*, 1996, 16, 412-24.

[7] Mandel, NS; Mandel, GS. Urinary tract stone disease in the United States veteran population. II. Geographical analysis of variations in composition. *The Journal of urology*, 1989, 142, 1516-21.

[8] Lieske, JC; Pena, de, la, Vega, LS; Slezak, JM; et, al. Renal stone epidemiology in Rochester, Minnesota: an update. *Kidney international*, 2006, 69, 760-4.

[9] Shekarriz, B; Stoller, ML. Uric acid nephrolithiasis: current concepts and controversies. *The Journal of urology*, 2002, 168, 1307-14.

[10] Pak, CY; Hayashi, Y; Arnold, LH. Heterogeneous nucleation with urate, calcium phosphate and calcium oxalate. Proceedings of the Society for Experimental Biology and Medicine Society for Experimental Biology and Medicine (New York, NY), 1976, 153, 83-7.

[11] Wu, XW; Muzny, DM; Lee, CC; Caskey, CT. Two independent mutational events in the loss of urate oxidase during hominoid evolution. *Journal of molecular evolution*, 1992, 34, 78-84.

[12] Pak, CY; Sakhaee, K; Peterson, RD; Poindexter, JR; Frawley, WH. Biochemical profile of idiopathic uric acid nephrolithiasis. *Kidney international*, 2001, 60, 757-61.

[13] Sakhaee, K; Adams-Huet, B; Moe, OW; Pak, CY. Pathophysiologic basis for normouricosuric uric acid nephrolithiasis. *Kidney international*, 2002, 62, 971-9.

[14] Reddy, ST; Wang, CY; Sakhaee, K; Brinkley, L; Pak, CY. Effect of low-carbohydrate high-protein diets on acid-base balance, stone-forming propensity, and calcium metabolism. *American journal of kidney diseases: the official journal of the National Kidney Foundation*, 2002, 40, 265-74.

[15] Gonzalez-Senac, NM; Bailen, R; Torres, RJ; de Miguel, E; Puig, JG. Metabolic syndrome in primary gout. *Nucleosides, nucleotides & nucleic acids*, 2014, 33, 185-91.

[16] Pak, CY; Sakhaee, K; Moe, O; et al. Biochemical profile of stone-forming patients with diabetes mellitus. *Urology*, 2003, 61, 523-7.

[17] Daudon, M; Traxer, O; Conort, P; Lacour, B; Jungers, P. Type 2 diabetes increases the risk for uric acid stones. *Journal of the American Society of Nephrology: JASN*, 2006, 17, 2026-33.

[18] Daudon, M; Lacour, B; Jungers, P. Influence of body size on urinary stone composition in men and women. *Urological research*, 2006, 34, 193-9.

[19] Ekeruo, WO; Tan, YH; Young, MD; et al. Metabolic risk factors and the impact of medical therapy on the management of nephrolithiasis in obese patients. *The Journal of urology*, 2004, 172, 159-63.

[20] Kohjimoto, Y; Sasaki, Y; Iguchi, M; Matsumura, N; Inagaki, T; Hara, I. Association of metabolic syndrome traits and severity of kidney stones: results from a nationwide survey on urolithiasis in Japan. *American journal of kidney diseases: the official journal of the National Kidney Foundation*, 2013, 61, 923-9.

[21] Cho, ST; Jung, SI; Myung, SC; Kim, TH. Correlation of metabolic syndrome with urinary stone composition. *International journal of urology: official journal of the Japanese Urological Association*, 2013, 20, 208-13.

[22] Weiner, ID; Verlander, JW. Role of NH3 and NH4+ transporters in renal acid-base transport. *American journal of physiology Renal physiology*, 2011, 300, F11-23.

[23] Klisic, J; Hu, MC; Nief, V; et al. Insulin activates Na(+)/H(+) exchanger 3: biphasic response and glucocorticoid dependence. *American journal of physiology Renal physiology*, 2002, 283, F532-9.

[24] Abate, N; Chandalia, M; Cabo-Chan, AV, Jr; Moe, OW; Sakhaee, K. The metabolic syndrome and uric acid nephrolithiasis: novel features of renal manifestation of insulin resistance. *Kidney international*, 2004, 65, 386-92.

[25] Torres, RJ; Puig, JG; Jinnah, HA. Update on the phenotypic spectrum of Lesch-Nyhan disease and its attenuated variants. *Current rheumatology reports*, 2012, 14, 189-94.

[26] Gutman, AB; Yue, TF. URINARY AMMONIUM EXCRETION IN PRIMARY GOUT. *The Journal of clinical investigation*, 1965, 44, 1474-81.

[27] Burnier, M; Roch-Ramel, F; Brunner, HR. Renal effects of angiotensin II receptor blockade in normotensive subjects. *Kidney international*, 1996, 49, 1787-90.

[28] Lee, SJ; Terkeltaub, RA. New developments in clinically relevant mechanisms and treatment of hyperuricemia. *Current rheumatology reports*, 2006, 8, 224-30.

[29] Manuel, MA; Steele, TH. Changes in renal urate handling after prolonged thiazide treatment. *The American journal of medicine*, 1974, 57, 741-6.

[30] Jou, YC; Fang, CY; Chen, SY; et al. Proteomic study of renal uric acid stone. *Urology*, 2012, 80, 260-6.

[31] Boyce, WH. Organic matrix of human urinary concretions. *The American journal of medicine*, 1968, 45, 673-83.

[32] Aggarwal, KP; Narula, S; Kakkar, M; Tandon, C. Nephrolithiasis: molecular mechanism of renal stone formation and the critical role played by modulators. *BioMed research international*, 2013, 2013, 292953.

[33] Kavanagh, JP. Supersaturation and renal precipitation: the key to stone formation? *Urological research*, 2006, 34, 81-5.

[34] Babić-Ivančić, V; Füredi-Milhofer, H; Brown, WE; Gregory, TM. Precipitation diagrams and solubility of uric acid dihydrate. *Journal of Crystal Growth*, 1987, 83, 581-7.

[35] Kobayashi, T; Nishizawa, K; Mitsumori, K; Ogura, K. Impact of date of onset on the absence of hematuria in patients with acute renal colic. *The Journal of urology*, 2003, 170, 1093-6.

[36] Smith-Bindman, R; Aubin, C; Bailitz, J; et al. Ultrasonography versus computed tomography for suspected nephrolithiasis. *The New England journal of medicine*, 2014, 371, 1100-10.

[37] Fulgham, PF; Assimos, DG; Pearle, MS; Preminger, GM. Clinical effectiveness protocols for imaging in the management of ureteral calculous disease: AUA technology assessment. *The Journal of urology*, 2013, 189, 1203-13.

[38] Tack, D; Sourtzis, S; Delpierre, I; de Maertelaer, V; Gevenois, PA. Low-dose unenhanced multidetector CT of patients with suspected renal colic. *AJR American journal of roentgenology*, 2003, 180, 305-11.

[39] Ciaschini, MW; Remer, EM; Baker, ME; Lieber, M; Herts, BR. Urinary calculi: radiation dose reduction of 50% and 75% at CT--effect on sensitivity. Radiology, 2009, 251, 105-11.

[40] Horowitz, E; Schmidt, JD. Renal calculi in pregnancy. *Clinical obstetrics and gynecology*, 1985, 28, 324-38.

[41] Patel, SJ; Reede, DL; Katz, DS; Subramaniam, R; Amorosa, JK. Imaging the pregnant patient for nonobstetric conditions: algorithms and

radiation dose considerations. Radiographics: a review publication of the Radiological Society of North America, Inc, 2007, 27, 1705-22.

[42] Masselli, G; Derme, M; Bernieri, MG; et al. Stone disease in pregnancy: imaging-guided therapy. *Insights into imaging*, 2014.

[43] Liebman, SE; Taylor, JG; Bushinsky, DA. Uric acid nephrolithiasis. *Current rheumatology reports*, 2007, 9, 251-7.

[44] Sterrett, SP; Penniston, KL; Wolf, JS, Jr; Nakada, SY. Acetazolamide is an effective adjunct for urinary alkalization in patients with uric acid and cystine stone formation recalcitrant to potassium citrate. *Urology*, 2008, 72, 278-81.

[45] Odvina, CV. Comparative value of orange juice versus lemonade in reducing stone-forming risk. *Clinical journal of the American Society of Nephrology: CJASN*, 2006, 1, 1269-74.

[46] Kang, DE; Sur, RL; Haleblian, GE; Fitzsimons, NJ; Borawski, KM; Preminger, GM. Long-term lemonade based dietary manipulation in patients with hypocitraturic nephrolithiasis. *The Journal of urology*, 2007, 177, 1358-62, discussion 62, quiz 591.

[47] Dretler, SP; Pfister, RC. Percutaneous dissolution of renal calculi. *Annual review of medicine*, 1983, 34, 359-66.

[48] Pfister, RC; Dretler, SP. Percutaneous chemolysis of renal calculi. *Urologic radiology*, 1984, 6, 138-43.

[49] Krenitsky, TA; Elion, GB; Strelitz, RA; Hitchings, GH. Ribonucleosides of allopurinol and oxoallopurinol. Isolation from human urine, enzymatic synthesis, and characterization. *The Journal of biological chemistry*, 1967, 242, 2675-82.

[50] Simmonds, HA; Reiter, S; Davies, PM; Cameron, JS. Orotidine accumulation in human erythrocytes during allopurinol therapy: association with high urinary oxypurinol-7-riboside concentrations in renal failure and in the Lesch-Nyhan syndrome. *Clinical science*, (London, England: 1979), 1991, 80, 191-7.

[51] Kamatani, N; Fujimori, S; Hada, T; et al. An allopurinol-controlled, randomized, double-dummy, double-blind, parallel between-group, comparative study of febuxostat (TMX-67), a non-purine-selective inhibitor of xanthine oxidase, in patients with hyperuricemia including those with gout in Japan: phase 3 clinical study. *Journal of clinical rheumatology: practical reports on rheumatic & musculoskeletal diseases*, 2011, 17, S13-8.

[52] Becker, MA; Schumacher, HR, Jr; Wortmann, RL; et al. Febuxostat compared with allopurinol in patients with hyperuricemia and gout. *The New England journal of medicine*, 2005, 353, 2450-61.

[53] Stamp, LK. Safety profile of anti-gout agents: an update. *Current opinion in rheumatology*, 2014, 26, 162-8.

[54] Hande, KR; Noone, RM; Stone, WJ. Severe allopurinol toxicity. Description and guidelines for prevention in patients with renal insufficiency. *The American journal of medicine*, 1984, 76, 47-56.

[55] Zagone, RL; Waldmann, TM; Conlin, MJ. Fragmentation of uric acid calculi with the holmium: YAG laser produces cyanide. *Lasers in surgery and medicine*, 2002, 31, 230-2.

In: Nephrolithiasis
Editor: Melody Shneider

ISBN: 978-1-63482-134-6

Chapter III

The Role of Ureteroscopy in the Management of Urolithiasis

Peter Tsambarlis[1] John Richgels [2] Christopher Coogan [3] and Kalyan Latchamsetty[4]

[1]Rush University Medical Center, Chicago, Illinois, US
[2]Rush Medical College, Chicago, Illinois, US
[3]Rush University Medical Center, Chicago, Illinois, US
[4]Rush University Medical Center, Chicago, Illinois, US

Abstract

Purpose: The aim of this review is to examine the utility of ureteroscopy in the management of ureteral stones.

Introduction: Throughout ureteroscopy's relatively brief history, clinical utility has paralleled technological advancement. This review follows that progression beginning with Dr. Young's placement of a pediatric cystoscope into a child's dilated ureter.

Technique: The method for both rigid and flexible ureteroscopy is discussed. We will also review potential pitfalls and discuss techniques that can help avoid potential complications. Finally, the debate on the use of ureteral stents during ureteroscopy is examined.

Results: Although the efficacy of ureteroscopy is well documented, this review pays particular attention to factors which influence stone free rates and how to maximize success. Risk factors for complications are identified and techniques proposed to achieve the highest possible success rates based on expert experience.

Discussion: Ureteroscopy is a safe and effective option for management of ureteral stones. Using the techniques described here, stone free rates are extremely high and risk is minimized. Furthermore, with the decreasing size of ureteroscopic instruments and improving images, complication rates should continue to decline.

Keywords: urolithiasis, flexible ureteroscopy, rigid ureteroscopy, laser lithotripsy

Introduction

History

Ureteroscopy can trace its beginnings back to renowned urological pioneer Hugh Hampton Young, when in 1912 he inadvertently advanced a pediatric cystoscope into the dilated ureter of a child with posterior urethral valves. Direct visualization of the renal pelvis for the first time opened the door to new therapeutic and diagnostic modalities that would permanently alter the practice of urology. Unfortunately, Young's advancement did not receive widespread recognition until his experience was published in a review article concerning congenital valvular obstruction in 1929.

Despite the discovery of ureteroscopy using the equivalent of what would be eventually known as a rigid scope, the next advancement in ureteroscopy would come from the use of fiber optic technology in the form of flexible ureteroscopes. In fact, the first practical use of ureteroscopes was in patients with nephrolithiasis. In 1960, Marshall inserted a fiberoptic scope, which was developed by pioneering gastroenterologist Basil Hirschowitz, 5 centimeters below the renal pelvis to examine the ureter for renal calculi. Two years later, Marshall's colleagues, McGovern and Walzak, performed the first retrograde, transurethral ureteroscopy to visualize a ureteral stone. This retrograde technique is the standard methodology that is still used today.

Rigid ureteroscopy's evolution in clinical applications was delayed in comparison to its flexible counterpart. In 1977, Tobias Goodman published his experiences using a rigid 11F pediatric cystoscope. The rigid cystoscope was used in one patient to inspect the ureteropelvic junction for mechanical obstruction; in another patient a biopsy of irregular ureteral mucosa was obtained; in a third patient, the rigid cystoscope was used to fulgurate a ureteral tumor. While the use in these patients resulted in no major complications, Goodman could foresee future complications and mentions ureteral perforation and injury by force of the instrument as potential hazards that must be avoided with "greatest gentleness." Lyons described the use of a 13F pediatric cystoscope safely in both men and women. In women, ureteral dilation was performed using Jewitt sounds prior to insertion of the pediatric cystoscope. In men, however, a 25.5 F pediatric cystoscope was passed into the bladder followed by ureteral dilation which was subsequently followed by the 13F scope into the ureter. This technique is mirrored today with the use of ureteral access sheaths and helps to minimize the risk of perforations. Additionally, Lyons saw the future of endoscopy when he proposed that a 14.5F resectoscope could be paired with a pediatric cystoscope sheath in order to utilize coagulation tools or baskets to perform minimally invasive therapeutic procedures. This paralleled the first designed "ureteroscope" made by Richard Wolf Medical Instruments in 1979 with large enough sheaths for visualization and manipulation. This is an advantage that early rigid scopes had over their flexible counterparts.

As the clinical utility of ureteroscopes evolved, ureteroscopic instruments and tools were being developed for treating and diagnosing upper urinary tract pathology. As early as 1966, the use of lasers for treating upper tract tumors and stones was theorized and tested using animal models.

Throughout the 1970's Takayasu demonstrated the utility of flexible ureteroscopes with deflectable tips which allowed for a far superior range of vision for diagnosis and treatment. However, despite this enhanced ability to see further and record the findings, these flexible ureteroscopes had no irrigation or working channels for passing instruments and thus had limited therapeutic use.

The benefits of ureteroscopy for treating nephrolithiasis quickly became apparent as scope technology evolved. Before 1981, all stones were treated by open lithotomy, or through retrograde blind manipulation which had significant associated morbidity, until Das described the first stone extraction from the distal ureter using the pediatric cystoscope. Changes in scope engineering allowed for more and more effective utilization and novel uses. Karl Storz Endoscopy engineered a longer specialized "ureteroscope" that could reach the renal pelvis at 50 cm of length. This scope allowed for more accurate diagnostic procedures such as biopsies and also allowed direct viewing for procedures that involved stone or tissue manipulation. These scopes also utilized interchangeable lenses with varying degrees for optimal fields of view, differed in sizes from 9-16F, and most importantly, had a working 5F channel that could accommodate instruments such as forceps, coagulation tools, and stone baskets. Huffman et al. published the first papers describing the successful use of the new Storz rigid scope for diagnosing upper urinary tract tumors and extracting calculi while establishing its safety. Huffman also envisioned the potential use of these scopes paired with the obliterative power of lithotripsy, when he described the first use of an ultrasonic lithotripter. The stone was held in place by a basket while the telescoping lens was removed and the lithotripter put in its place. Contact between the device and stone was then confirmed by fluoroscopy. This technique's efficacy for stone removal and safety was further confirmed by the work of Green et al. who was able to perform the procedure under direct visualization. By 1985, clinical efficacy and safety of intraureteral management of urinary calculi had been established. This was largely due to the advancements in ureteroscope technology and the development of instruments for direct visualization and manipulation of calculi.

Lithotripsy for ureteral stones is simple enough in concept, however its clinical efficacy has been determined by the type of scope available for use (rigid vs flexible,) its potential for damaging human tissue, ease of use, and effectiveness. Ultrasonic and pneumatic devices have been in use since 1952 with high success rates. Their use, however, was only compatible with rigid scopes, which, therefore, limited their utility in treating upper urinary tract stones, and carried an increased risk of ureteral injury. Laser energy for stone fragmentation, however, was an attractive option because of the maximal burst of energy in a small, focused space which minimizes collateral tissue damage. Laser energy can also be transmitted along flexible fibers, which makes it ideal for use in flexible ureteroscopes that can reach and maneuver the lower calices. Pulsed dye lasers were initially used for lithotripsy in 1984, but the costs were high and the fragmentation of hard calcium oxalate stones was less than ideal. The Nd: YAG laser combined pulsed dye with infrared and was effective in minimizing damage to the ureter. However, it also had difficulty fragmenting hard stones. The Holmium (Ho: Yag) is a midinfrared laser which was first used in 1993 for lithotripsy. It was found to have ideal properties for fragmentation and tissue coagulation or fulguration to help treat stones, tumors, and strictures. Johnson et al. described the potential of this laser's small flexible fibers, ability to fragment calcium oxalate stones, and power selectivity for versatile clinical applications. Over the years, the Holmium laser has established an excellent efficacy and safety profile and is considered the leading method for intraureteral stone lithotripsy

Preoperative Considerations

Prior to proceeding to the operating room for a ureteroscopic procedure, all patients should undergo the standard preoperative workup. A CT scan is very helpful in operative planning and it will guide the approach based on the size and position of the calculus. It is also critical to rule out any active infection prior to performing ureteroscopy. Thus, a negative preoperative urine culture should be obtained before proceeding with definitive treatment. If the patient is febrile or has a urinalysis which is positive for infection we recommend stent placement followed by a full course of antibiotics prior to ureteroscopic management of the stones. The risks of performing ureteroscopy in an infected system and potentially causing bacteremia and sepsis outweigh the benefits of managing the stone quickly with a single procedure.

Techniques

Regardless of the type of ureteroscope used, the patient is positioned in the dorsal lithotomy position and prepped and draped in the standard sterile fashion. At our institution, general anesthesia is used for the vast majority of ureteroscopic cases.

Rigid Ureteroscopy

Initially the bladder is entered via a cystoscope and is thoroughly surveyed. Particular care should be placed on identifying any bladder stones that can be managed simultaneously. Any signs of infection should be noted that may alter the course of the operation if present. Ureteroscopy should not be undertaken in the setting of an active infection as previously noted. After a complete survey is performed, the ureteral orifices are identified. If a stent is present, it should be grasped with an alligator-toothed forceps and brought out to the meatus, taking care to minimize the amount the stent is manipulated. Ideally, the end of the stent should remain proximal to the stone so that a wire may be passed beyond the stone with minimal manipulation. This, however, can be quite challenging, particularly in a male patient with a proximal ureteral stone.

If a stent is not present at the time of ureteroscopy, the ureter can be cannulated directly with a wire. A number of different wires can be used to achieve this. In our experience, a Coons-Bentson wire is a good first choice due to its removable core. If the stone cannot be passed with a Coons-Bentson wire, a glidewire with or without the aid of a torque vice is an excellent alternative as it minimizes potential trauma to the ureter. If a glidewire is used to traverse the stone, it should be exchanged with an exchange catheter for a more firm wire, such as a Coons-Bentson wire, prior to proceeding.

Once the ureter is cannulated and the stone traversed, the wire is secured to the drape as a safety wire. The rigid ureteroscope is then inserted into the meatus and advanced into the bladder in the same fashion as a cystoscope being inserted under direct vision. The safety wire can be used as a guide to the ureteral orifice. If possible, the ureteroscope should be inserted under the safety wire up the ureter to the level of the stone. If any resistance is encountered, one should consider using a flexible ureteroscope instead of the rigid. Once at the level of the stone, there are a number of tools that can be used to help with stone lithotripsy and stone extraction. For example, in the setting of a solitary stone with a high risk of upward migration and no additional stones in the proximal ureter or kidney, there are devices available which can prevent proximal migration. They do so by creating a barrier above the level of the stone.

Typically, a holmium laser is used to pulverize the stone. Different settings can be used with the holmium laser, but the goal is a balance between breaking the stone and minimizing nearby tissue damage. The fiber is inserted into the working channel of the ureteroscope and brought into contact with the stone.

The most efficient destruction of the stone is from the outside in. Working along the edges of the stone produces dust that will easily pass on its own. Minimizing the number of fragments is important for efficiency because it minimizes the amount of basket extraction required at the end of the case. Once the stone is broken into small fragments, the largest ones are removed via an endoscopic basket and sent for stone analysis.

After the fragments have been removed, a ureteral stent can be placed under fluoroscopic guidance using the safety wire.

Flexible Ureteroscopy

The technique for lithotripsy with a flexible ureteroscope is very similar to the rigid ureteroscope. As previously described, the flexible ureteroscope is more useful for proximal and renal pelvic stones. It also carries a smaller risk of ureteral perforation.

The bladder is entered and the ureter is cannulated with a wire as described above with or without the aid of a stent. After placement of the initial wire, however, the procedure differs. The flexible ureteroscope can be passed directly or with the use of a ureteral access sheath. If using the sheath, it is carefully inserted up to, but not past, the ureteral calculus. Passing the ureteral access sheath beyond the level of the stone increases the risk of impaction into the side wall. A second wire is then placed through the ureteral access sheath and the sheath removed. One of the two wires is then secured to the drape as the safety wire. The ureteral access sheath is placed over the remaining wire to the level of the stone again. The wire which was used to place the ureteral access sheath is removed along with the inner core of the access sheath.

Once this setup is achieved the ureteroscope can be passed up to the level of the stone via the access sheath and lithotripsy may be undertaken in the same manner as described above for rigid ureteroscopy. Again, stone fragments are sent for analysis, and a stent may be left in place at the conclusion of the procedure.

Success Rates

Ureteroscopy is an extremely effective means of producing high stone free rates. The factor which most predicts successful ureteroscopic management of stones is location of the stone with distal stones being more likely to be completely removed than proximal stones. Stone free rates in the distal ureter ranged from 91-99% (Pearle et al. 2001, Sofer et al. 2002, Zeng et al. 2002, Aghamir et al. 2003, Sozen et al. 2003). This can be compared to lower, but still high, success rates of more proximal stones ranging from 82 to 97% (Lam et al. 2002, Sofer et al. 2002, Aghamir et al. 2003, Sozen et al. 2003, Fong et al. 2004, Wu et al. 2005). These high rates continue to climb with more recent studies showing increasing stone free rates. A large retrospective study at the Mayo clinic of 1000 ureteroscopies showed an overall stone free rate of 91.4% regardless of stone size or location (Krambeck et al. 2006). A more recent randomized controlled study of 200 patients revealed a total stone free rate of 88% compared to only 60% for ESWL. In this study, all stones were over 1 cm in size (Salem 2009).

Complications

There are numerous minor complications associated with ureteroscopy including pain, bleeding, and infections. Major complications, fortunately, are rare with this procedure. Two major intraoperative complications that have been described are avulsion and intussusception. Both of these complications are most commonly associated with placing excessive traction on a stone or stone fragment that is too large to traverse the ureter. Furthermore, the risk of both complications can be minimized by careful and sufficient lithotripsy. Two reviews demonstrate the decreasing frequency with which avulsion occurs. In a review of 33 series by Stoller and Wolf (1996) 17 out of 5117 patients had their ureteroscopy procedure complicated by an avulsion between 1984 and 1992. In a later review, however, 0 out of 1059 patients undergoing ureteroscopy for stone disease had an avulsion (Grasso 2001). Both intussusception and avulsion may require laparoscopic or open repair due to devitalization of the ureter. Therefore, although rare, it is important to keep both in mind when performing ureteroscopy.

Stricture is another complication of concern, thus often justifying the use of postoperative stenting. However, the incidence of stricture has been decreasing as scope sizes have decreased and techniques improved, with documented rates between 1-2% (Kijvikai 2007). Urinary tract infections and urosepsis are documented complications that can be associated with excessive flushing, increased operative times, and chronic UTI patients which can be of significant risk to patients. Urosepsis is a rare complication after ureteroscopy. The AUA 2007 guidelines report its occurrence in 2-4% of patients. More recently, the Endourologic Society's URS Global Study reported a urosepsis rate of 0.3% (de la Rosette 2014). However, given its severity, and the fact that a obtaining a negative urine culture in all patients is not always possible, the use of perioperative antibiotics in patients undergoing ureteroscopy is justified and recommended. There is also a risk of migration of the stone proximally in the ureter during the procedure which can result in longer operating times, more invasive endoscopy, and secondary procedures. The use of stone antiretropulsion devices, however, has decreased the incidence of this complication. Finally, if the patient's stone burden is not relieved, the patient is at risk for secondary procedures for definitive treatment. However, as previously described, stone-free rates for ureteroscopy have been steadily increasing as institutions gain more experience and as techniques continue to improve.

Stents and Ureteroscopy

There is some debate as to whether or not stents should be placed after ureteroscopy for management of stones. Ureteral injuries are often managed with stents and thus it has been held that they should be used during ureteroscopic manipulation of the GU tract. At our institution, stents are used in over 96% of cases. This is done because we hold that when the ureter is dilated, a stent is the most effective way to prevent post-operative obstruction. We use active dilation in most cases in the form of a ureteral access sheath. Likewise, when patients are stented prior to definitive management of the stone, one benefit is the passive dilation which results in easier access to the ureter when definitive management is undertaken. Furthermore, readmission rates have been shown to be lower in patients who are stented than patients who are not (Prodromos 2001).

There are arguments, however, against the routine use of ureteral stents. Some studies have shown patients who have undergone routine stent placement at the time of ureteroscopy experience more of the following: flank pain, urinary symptoms, bladder pain, overall pain, and narcotic use (Prodromos 2001, El Harrech 2014). Jeong on the other hand, did not find a difference in those measures but did see an increase in hematuria in the stented group (2004). These studies concluded that uncomplicated ureteroscopy without the use of ureteral dilation can be safely performed without the use of routine stenting. Despite this debate it is important to point out two absolute indications for stent placement. A stent should be placed any time stone management is undertaken in a solitary kidney or if any ureteral injury or perforation is suspected. We have found, if needed, that stent bother can be effectively managed by the use of Tamsulosin.

Conclusion

Ureteroscopy is a safe, effective option for management of ureteral stones. Using the techniques described in this review, stone free rates are comparable to, or superior to, all other methods of managing urolithiasis and continue to rise. Furthermore, with the decreasing size of ureteroscopic instruments and improving images with digital ureteroscopes, complication rates should continue to decline.

References

[1] Johnston el al 2004. W. Johnston III. R Low. S Das. The Evolution and Progress of Ureteroscopy. *Urologic Clinics of North America.* 31(1) Feb 2004.

[2] Goodman 1977. Goodman TM. Ureteroscopy with pediatric cystoscope in adults. *Urology* 1977;9(4):pp. 394.

[3] Young et al. 1929. Young HH, McKay RW. Congenital valve obstruction of the prostatic urethra. *Surg. Gynecol. Obstet.* 1929;48:pp. 509.

[4] Marshall 1964. Marshall VF. Fiberoptics in urology. *J. Urol.* 1964;(91) pp. 110-4.

[5] Takayasu et al. 1971. Takayasu H, Aso Y, Go T. Clinical application of fiberoptic pyeloureteroscope. *Urol. Int.* 1971;26: pp 97-104.

[6] Lyon et al. 1978. Lyon ES, Kyker JS, Schoenberg HW. Transurethral ureteroscopy in women: a ready addition to the urological armamentarium. *J. Urol.* 1978;119:pp. 35.

[7] Huffman et al. 1983. Huffman JL, Bagley DH, Lyon ES. Extending cystoscopic techniques into the ureter and renal pelvis. *JAMA* 1983; 250(15):2002.

[8] Green et al. 1985. Green DF, Lytton B. Early experience with direct vision electrohydraulic lithotripsy of ureteral calculi. *J. Urol.* 1985;133:767.

[9] Lee et al. 2009. Lee J,_Gianduzzo TR. Advances in laser technology in urology. *Urol. Clin. North Am.* 2009 May;36(2): pp. 189-98,

[10] Johnson et al. 1992. Johnson DE, Cromeens DM, Price RE. Use of the holmium:YAG laser in urology. *Lasers Surg. Med.* 1992;12: pp. 353-63.

[11] Pearle et al, 2001. Pearle MS, Nadler R, Bercowsky E, et al: Prospective randomized trial comparing shock wave lithotripsy and ureteroscopy for management of distal ureteral calculi. *J. Urol.* 2001; 166: pp. 1255-1260.

[12] Sofer et al, 2002. Sofer M, Watterson JD, Wollin TA, et al: Holmium:yag laser lithotripsy for upper urinary tract calculi in 598 patients. *J. Urol.* 2002; 167: pp. 31-34.

[13] Zeng et al, 2002. Zeng GQ, Zhong WD, Cai YB, et al: Extracorporeal shock wave versus pneumatic ureteroscopic lithotripsy in treatment of lower ureteral calculi. *Asian J. Androl.* 2002; 4: pp. 303-305.

[14] Aghamir, Mohseni, Ardestani, 2003. Aghamir SK, Mohseni MG, and Ardestani A: Treatment of ureteral calculi with ballistic lithotripsy. *J. Endourol.* 2003; 17: pp. 887-890.

[15] Sozen et al, 2003. Sozen S, Kupeli B, Tunc L, et al: Management of ureteral stones with pneumatic lithotripsy: report of 500 patients. *J. Endourol.* 2003; 17: pp. 721-724.

[16] Lam, Greene, Gupta, 2002. Lam JS, Greene TD, and Gupta M: Treatment of proximal ureteral calculi: holmium:YAG laser ureterolithotripsy versus extracorporeal shock wave lithotripsy. *J. Urol.* 2002; 167: pp. 1972-1976.

[17] Fong et al, 2004. Fong YK, Ho SH, Peh OH, et al: Extracorporeal shockwave lithotripsy and intracorporeal lithotripsy for proximal ureteric calculi—a comparative assessment of efficacy and safety. *Ann. Acad. Med. Singapore* 2004; 33: pp. 80-83.

[18] Wu et al, 2005. Wu CF, Chen CS, Lin WY, et al: Therapeutic options for proximal ureter stone: extracorporeal shock wave lithotripsy versus semirigid ureterorenoscope with holmium:yttrium aluminum garnet laser lithotripsy. *Urology* 2005; 65: pp. 1075-1079.

[19] Krambeck et al, 2006. Murat FJ, Gettman MT, Chow GK, Patterson DE, Segura JW: The evolution of ureteroscopy: a modern single-institution series. *Mayo Clin. Proc.* 2006;81(4): pp. 468.

[20] Salem 2009. Salem HK: A prospective randomized study comparing shock wave lithotripsy and semirigid ureteroscopy for the management of proximal ureteral calculi. *Urology.* 2009;74(6): pp. 1216a.

[21] Stoller et al. 1996. Stoller ML and Wolf JS. Endoscopic ureteral injuries. In:McAninch JW, editor. Traumatic and reconstructive urology. Philadelphia: WB Saunders; 1996. pp. 199-211.8.

[22] Grasso M. Complications of ureteropyloscopy.In: Taneja SS, Smith RB, Ehrlich RM, editors.Complications of urologic surgery. 3rd edition.Philadelphia: WB Saunders; 2001. pp. 268-76.
[23] K Kijvikai et al. 2007. Kijvikai K, Haleblian GE. Preminger GM. de la Rosette J. Shock wave lithotripsy or ureteroscopy for the management of proximal ureteral calculi; an old discussion revisited. *J. Urol.* 2007;178: pp. 1157-63.
[24] Preminger et al. 2007. Preminger GM, Tiselius HG, Assimos DG, Alken P, Buck C, Gallucci M, Knoll T, Lingeman JE, Nakada SY, Pearle MS, Sarica K, Türk C, Wolf JS Jr; EAU/AUA Nephrolithiasis Guideline Panel. 2007 guidelines for the management of ureteral calculi. *The Journal of Urology*. 2007 Dec;178(6):2418-34.
[25] de la Rosette et al. 2014. de la Rosette Jean, Denstedt John, Geavlete Petrisor, Keeley Francis, Matsuda Tadashi, Pearle Margaret, Preminger Glenn, Traxer Olivier, and on behalf of the CROES URS Study Group. *Journal of Endourology*. February 2014, 28(2): 131-139.
[26] Prodromos et al. 2001 Prodromos BG, Amling, Schenkman NS Manoj M, Ward JF, Piper NY, Bishoff JT, Kane CJ: Ureteral Stenting After Ureteroscopy for Distal Ureteral Calculi: A Multi-Institutional Prospective Randomized Controlled Study Assessing Pain, Outcomes, and Complications. *J. Urol.* 2001; 166: pp. 1651-1657.
[27] El Harrech Et al. 2014. El Harrech Y, Abakka N, El Anzaoui J, Ghoundale O, Touiti D. Ureteral Stenting after Uncomplicated Ureteroscopy for Distal Ureteral Stones: A Randomized, Controlled Trial. *Minimally Invasive Surgery* 2014;2014:892890.
[28] Jeong H et al. 2004. Jeong H, Kwak C, Lee SE. Ureteric stenting after ureteroscopy for ureteric stones: a prospective randomized study assessing symptoms and complications. *BJU Int.* 2004 May;93(7): pp. 1032-4.

In: Nephrolithiasis
Editor: Melody Shneider

ISBN: 978-1-63482-134-6

Chapter IV

Renal Calcium and Urate Handling and Diet in Idiopathic Calcium Stone Formers

***Valerie Walker*[1*] *and Damian G. Griffin*[2]**
[1]Department of Clinical Biochemistry, University Hospital Southampton NHS Foundation Trust, Southampton, UK
[2]Department of Clinical Biochemistry, Galway University Hospital, Galway, Republic of Ireland

Abstract

The incidence of calcium stones is increasing world-wide. Dietary changes which impact on urine composition are probably largely responsible. However, despite years of research, we still do not have a clear understanding of the underlying defects in hypercalciuria or hyperuricosuria in idiopathic calcium stone formers or of how diet is implicated. Without this, interventions to prevent stone recurrence are largely empirical and often biased by personal opinion.

From our own stone clinic we reported that male stone formers with idiopathic hypercalciuria reabsorb less of the calcium filtered into the

* Corresponding Author: Department of Clinical Biochemistry, C Level MP6, South Block, Southampton General Hospital, Tremona Road, Southampton SO16 6YD, UK Tel +44 2381 206436. valerie.walker@uhs.nhs.uk.

kidneys than men with normocalciuria. Similarly, net urate reabsorption of men with idiopathic hyperuricosuria is reduced compared with those with normal urate excretion. This is probably explained by genetic variation in the renal transport of calcium and urate in the general population. In an earlier study, in which we investigated families in which three or more first degree relatives had stones, we confirmed the heritability of hypercalciuria. From our growing knowledge of the numerous genes which are implicated in the renal handling of calcium and urate, and of their close interaction, genetic variation is inevitable. There is increasing interest in this area, but so far few associations have been identified between genetic polymorphisms of renal transporters and hypercalciuria or hyperuricosuria.

From our clinic, we also found subsets of male stone formers with hypercalciuria and hyperuricosuria who had very high creatinine clearance rates, and hence (by inference) glomerular filtration rates. This would lead to delivery of an abnormally high filtered load of calcium or urate to the kidneys. We do not know the explanation. However, one possibility is a high dietary protein intake. There is a large body of evidence that high intakes increase glomerular filtration. From recent studies this might be mediated by enhanced nitric oxide production via the renal arginine-citrulline cycle, which could also influence intrarenal blood flow. This merits further exploration.

As in the case of hypercholesterolemia, idiopathic hypercalciuria and uricosuria may result from interaction between increased genetic susceptibility and dietary excesses, particularly of protein. Whilst identification of those with unfavorable diets and appropriate intervention should reduce calcium or urate excretion of hypercalciuric and hyperuricosuric stone formers, it will not be enough for those at the more severe end of the spectrum for genetic abnormality. They will need additional medication which, hopefully, may be targeted towards specific transporters in the future. With the advances in the technology for rapid through-put DNA analysis, we now have the opportunity to get to the roots of the problem, but it will be fundamental to define the phenotypes of stone formers as precisely as possible if the genetic analyses are to be fruitful.

Introduction

Stones are a common problem world-wide and occur 2-4 times more often in men than women. In America, the life-time risk for stones for men is 12% and for women 5% [1] with estimated annual incidences for men ranging from 100 to 300 per 100,000. [2] Their prevalence has risen over the last 40 years.

[3-5] There is a high recurrence rate, estimated at around 25% at 10y for a first time stone former and 75% for recurrent stone formers. [6] The evidence that hypercalciuria is more common among idiopathic calcium stone formers than in the general population, and that it increases the risk for renal stones is beyond doubt. Precise definition is impossible because urinary calcium excretion is a continuous variable, but using commonly adopted thresholds for urine calcium of >7.50 mmol/24h for men and > 6.25 mmol/24h for women [1], 30- 50% of adult stone-formers have hypercalciuria [3, 7, 8] compared with fewer than 10% in the general population. [3] The underlying cause of hypercalciuria has been investigated intensively. Intestinal calcium absorption is increased, but negative calcium balance develops with dietary calcium restriction which indicates impaired renal conservation of calcium ('renal hypercalciuria') together with increased mobilization of calcium from bone ('resorptive hypercalciuria'). Formerly, patients with idiopathic hypercalciuria were classified as having absorptive, renal or resorptive hypercalciuria and this directed their management. [7-9] However, this categorization was difficult in a clinic setting and interpretation of calcium loading tests used in research clinics to demonstrate absorptive hypercalciuria [10] may have been confounded by co-existing renal hypercalciuria. Indeed, it was suggested that all idiopathic hypercalciuria may be in part renal. [11] In experimental studies on a genetic stone-forming rat all three mechanisms contribute to hypercalciuria, [12] and there is a growing consensus that this is also the case in humans. [1, 3, 8, 9, 13-15] Pedigree and twin studies have demonstrated that hypercalciuria is inherited, with the genetic contribution to urinary excretion estimated at around 50%. [4, 16-20] The heritability of this quantitative trait is polygenic in nature. [15, 18, 19]

Fewer than 20% of individuals with hypercalciuria in the general population have symptomatic stone disease. [7] Hypercalciuria may merely lower the threshold for urolithiasis which is then triggered by other associated factors, such as low urine volume, abnormal urinary pH, and excessive oxalate or urate excretion. These could have a genetic origin and/or result from environmental factors, particularly low fluid intake and diet. They must be controlled in addition to hypercalciuria if interventions to reduce stone recurrence are to be effective. [3, 8]

In view of the numerous variables which may contribute to 'idiopathic' hypercalciuria, investigations to further our understanding of its origin and significance for stone formation must be targeted. We need to identify sub-groups of patients for study who have a homogeneous phenotype with an increased likelihood of having a selected pathological defect.

In this chapter we report findings from our own clinic in Southampton. In an early family study we looked for evidence of linkage between stone formation and intermediate traits associated with stones with four genes which are involved in calcium turnover. The findings have not been previously reported and will be covered in detail. In our other studies we aimed to identify patients from the clinic data base whose predominant abnormality was low renal calcium or urate reabsorption and to look for associated risks for stones. The main findings of three studies which have been published [21-23] will be summarized. Collectively they support the case for a genetic contribution to hypercalciuria, hyperuricosuria and stones in some families, indicate that altered renal tubular handling of calcium and urate is probably a common underlying factor in hypercalciuria and hyperuricosuria, that individuals in whom this is the dominant primary abnormality can be identified in a clinic setting and that their risk factors for stones differ from those of individuals whose dominant disturbance is delivery of an excessive filtered load of calcium or urate to the kidney.

The Southampton Stone Clinic

The Renal Stone Clinic of the Department of Clinical Biochemistry at Southampton General Hospital UK accepts referrals for stone forming patients diagnosed in the local area. Its purpose is to identify and treat factors which can be modified to reduce the risk of stone recurrence. A clinic database, held on Microsoft Access (97-2003), was created in 1996 and includes demographic and biochemical data for most patients investigated for stones who initially presented to the Clinic between June 1990 and March 2007. [21] The data were anonymized for the research studies. At the first attendance, non-fasting blood and a paired fresh random urine sample were collected. With careful verbal and written instruction, patients collected 24h urine samples at home, without refrigeration. From around 1997, patients collected one 24h sample with thymol as preservative. On receipt, the volume was determined from weight and an aliquot was removed for urate analysis without pH adjustment. The urine remaining in the container was then acidified with hydrochloric acid to pH 2.0. Prior to 1997, patients collected two samples: one into hydrochloric acid for the standard tests, and the second into sodium hydroxide for urate analysis if requested. The pH was then adjusted to 2.0 and 7.5, respectively.

The standard tests were: plasma: electrolytes, bicarbonate, creatinine, calcium adjusted for albumin, phosphate, urate and parathyroid hormone (PTH); fresh random urine: pH, phosphate and creatinine concentrations; 24h urine: volume, calcium, oxalate, creatinine and creatinine clearance. 24h urine urate, citrate and magnesium were added variably, often for patients with more severe stone problems. All analyses were carried out at Southampton General Hospital. Stones were analyzed qualitatively, with chemical methods using a Merckognost urinary calculi analysis kit (Merck, Darmstadt, Germany). Non-parametric statistical analyses were used throughout: the two-tailed Mann-Whitney U test and two-sided Fisher's exact test or Chi-square tests to compare differences between groups and Spearman's rank test for correlation.

The Family Study

This study was undertaken between 1997 and 2000. From the clinic database, 25 patients were selected who were recorded as having at least two first-degree relatives with renal stone disease. Selection was biased towards families with young index patients (more likely to have a severe defect and living relatives), affected women (lower incidence of stones than men and possibly a greater likelihood of having a genetic defect), and those living locally. Families of index patients with a known heritable cause of nephrolithiasis were excluded. Fourteen families were finally recruited and participants gave written informed consent. All participants who lived locally provided a blood sample for biochemistry and DNA extraction, a mouthwash for DNA, and fasting and 24h urine samples. Adults living outside Southampton provided a mouthwash sample, fasting urine and if possible, blood for DNA collected locally. Children under 16 years of age provided a mouthwash sample and fasting urine.

To explore the familial basis of renal stone disease, the heritability of stones and relevant biochemical traits were inspected for each kindred. The possibility that these were linked to any of four genes which might be implicated in stone disease was investigated using a microsatellite-based approach for co-segregation analysis. The microsatellite markers were tetranucleotide repeats with between 5 and 9 alleles and heterozygosity frequencies $\geq$ 60%. The selected genes were those for the calcium sensing receptor (CASR; location 3q21-q24), the thiazide-sensitive sodium chloride cotransporter (SLC34A1; 16q13), vitamin D receptor (12q12-q14), and the sodium–phosphate cotransporter (NPT2; 5q35). Genehunter, a software program that facilitates non-parametric linkage analysis, was used to analyze for linkage between renal stone affection status and the genotyped microsatellite markers in 14 pedigrees. BETA, a software program that facilitates non-parametric linkage analysis for a quantitative trait using allele sharing in sibling pairs, was used to analyze for linkage between quantitative traits associated with renal stone disease and the genotyped microsatellite markers. A LOD score $\approx$ 3.0, approximates to a significance level of 5% for Mendelian disorders.

Summary of the Findings

Biochemical analyses were undertaken on samples from 14 kindreds from 166 individuals $\geq$ 18 years of age and 34 aged <18 years. The key relevant data for each family are summarized in Table 1. Samples were obtained for 10 or more members of seven families, but other families were smaller with few surviving members living locally to recruit.

Hypercalciuria

Overall, 32 of 105 individuals (30%) who supplied 24h urine samples had hypercalciuria. The incidence was significantly higher in stone formers than in non-stone formers (45% versus 22%, P 0.016). The frequency varied among the families and was apparently a common abnormality in four of the larger kindreds tested (1, 2, 10, and 11), and possibly important in two other families (13, 14) in each of which two of the only three members tested were hypercalciuric. Hypercalciuria was relatively modest, with median values for men of 9.19 mmol/24h and for women of 7.50 mmol/24h, and only 7 individuals had values > 10.00 mmol /24h. Only 14% of adults had raised fasting urine calcium/creatinine ratios, with no difference between stone formers and non-stone formers, and no apparent segregation with the hypercalciuric kindreds. None of those under 18 years of age had had stones, but four (12%) had raised calcium/creatinine ratios.

Table 1. Abnormal findings in families of 14 stone formers with two or more first degree relatives with stones

Family (no. of stone formers tested)	Inc. 24h calcium (no. with stones)	†n	Inc. Ca/crt ratio (no. with stones)	n	<18y with inc Ca/crt (no. with stones)	n	Inc. 24h oxalate (no. with stones)	n	Low 24h citrate (no. with stones)	n	Low cit/crt ratio (no. with stones)	n	<18y with low cit/crt (no. with stones)	n	TmPO4 < 0.80 mmol/l (no. with stones)	n	Inc. 1,25-DHCC (no. with stones)	n	Inc. PTH (no. with stones)	n
1 (4)	4 (3)	9	2(1)	14	0	6	3(2)	9	0	9	3(0)	14	0	6	6(4)	8	3(0)	9	1(1)	9
2 (3)	6 (1)	10	7(1)	17	1	1	2(0)	10	1(1)	10	4(1)	16	1	1	2(1)	9	4(1)	6	0	9
3 (4)	1 (1*)	4	1(1*)	5	0	2	0	4	0	4	1(1)	5	0	2	3(3*)	4	0	4	1(1*)	4
4 (3)	1 (1*)	4	1(1*)	4	1	3	0	4	1(1*)	4	2(1)	4	0	3	2(1*)	4	3(2*)	4	1(1*)	4
5 (2)	0	3	0	5	none tested		0	3	0	3	1(0)	5	none tested		0	2	2(2)	3	0	3
6 (3)	1 (0)	13	2(0)	17	1	6	2(0)	13	0	13	3(1)	17	0	6	5(2)	12	2(0)	11	2(1)	12
7 (2)	0	6	0	8	none tested		1(0)	6	1(0)	6	2(1)	7	none tested		3(2)	5	3(2)	5	0	5
8 (2)	1 (1)	2	1(0)	5	0	1	0	2	0	2	2(1)	5	0	2	2(2)	2	1(1)	2	0	2
9 (1)	1 (1)	4	0	4	none tested		0	4	1(0)	4	2(0)	4	none tested		0	3	2(0)	4	0	4
10 (5)	4 (2)	7	2(1)	9	1	2	1(1)	7	1(1)	7	4(1)	10	0	2	1(1)	8	5(3)	8	0	8
11 (3)	5 (2)	10	2(0)	16	0	3	3(0)	10	2(0)	10	2(0)	17	0	3	2(1)	9	5(2)	9	1(0)	9
12 (5)	4 (3)	27	4(1)	39	0	6	3(0)	27	6(1)	25	**16(1)	39	2	6	4 (2)	17	6(3)	27	2(0)	25
13 (3)	2 (1)	3	2(1)	11	0	1	2(1)	3	2(1)	3	4(2)	11	1	1	2(1)	3	2(1)	3	0	3
14 (3)	2 (2)	3	0	8	0	2	0	3	0	3	2(1)	7	1	2	1(1)	3	0	3	0	3
Totals: abnorm (tested)																				
sf	18(40) 45%		7(41) 17%				4(40)10%		5(40) 13%		11(42) 26%				21(39) 54%		17(38) 45%		4 (40) 10%	
non-sf	14(65) 22%		17(125)14%		4 (33) 12%		13 (65) 20%		10(63) 16%		36(119)30%		5(34) 15%		12(50) 24%		21(60) 35%		4(60) 7%	
all	32(105)30%		24(166)14%				17(105)16%		15(103)15%		47(161)29%				33(89) 41%		38(98) 39%		8(100) 8%	

† Number of samples analyzed; * Results indicated that this stone former had primary hyperparathyroidism; ** 10 members of this kindred had fasting citrate/creatinine ratios < 0.10 mmol/mmol (ref ≥ 0.16); ref for calcium/ creatinine ratio for adults ≤ 0.59 mmol/mmol; <18years ≤ 0.69 mmol/mmol; Abbreviations: inc. increased; Ca/crt urine calcium/creatinine ratio; cit/creat: citrate/creatinine ratio; 1,25-DHCC 1,25-dihydroxycholecalciferol; PTH parathyroid hormone; sf stone formers; non-sf non-stone formers.

Table 2. Comparison of data for all adults ≥ 18 y with hypercalciuria (men urine calcium > 7.50 mmol/24h; women > 6.25 mmol/24h) with those with normocalciuria†

	MEN 24h calcium > 7.50 mmol median; range (n)	**MEN** 24h calcium ≤ 7.50 mmol median; range (n)	P†† high v normal	**WOMEN** 24h calcium > 6.25 mmol median; range (n)	**WOMEN**24h calcium ≤ 6.25 mmol median; range (n)	P high v normal
Total in group	16	33		13	40	
stones	11 (69%)	14 (42%)	0.128	6 (46%)	8 (20%)	0.030
Plasma						
Calcium mmol/l	2.41; 2.25-2.54 (15)	2.36; 2.24-2.61 (30)	0.288	2.32; 2.22-2.52 (13)	2.36; 2.20-2.59 (38)	0.043
Phosphate mmol/l	1.03; 0.71-1.38 (15)	1.02; 0.80-1.68 (30)	0.399	1.00; 0.80-1.27 (13)	1.14; 0.71-1.40 (38)	0.230
PTH pmol/l	3.3; 1.4-15.8 (15)	3.3; 1.1-10.6 (30)	0.952	3.1; 1.1-7.6 (13)	2.7; 0.6-8.1 (38)	0.762
1,25 DHCC pmol/l	120; 61-161 (15)	85; 46-182 (30)	0.044	126; 70-180 (13)	98; 38-151 (36)	0.029
24h urine						
Oxalate mmol/24h	0.46; 0.29-0.67 (16)	0.33; 0.12-0.67 (33)	0.002	0.36; 0.23-0.76 (13)	0.32; 0.14-0.94 (40)	0.121
Calcium mmol/24h	9.19; 7.53-16.81 (16)	5.24; 1.38-7.50 (33)	<0.001	7.50; 6.44-18.58 (13)	3.32; 1.17-6.24 (40)	<0.001
Citrate mmol/24h	4.06; 1.10-8.49 (16)	2.59; 3.77-21.92 (32)	0.018	3.48; 1.72-7.19 (13)	2.77; 0.35-5.74 (39)	0.148
Volume l/24h	1.83; 1.28-3.02 (16)	1.53; 0.78-2.65 (33)	0.002	1.69; 0.76-3.44 (13)	1.49; 0.49-3.91 (40)	0.347
Creatinine mmol/24h	15.9; 9.5-21.2 (16)	12.4; 3.8-21.9 (33)	0.001	12.6; 8.11-21.67 (13)	8.72; 3.6-16.0 (40)	0.002
Creatinine clearance l/24h	178; 70-263 (15)	125; 36-274 (30)	0.003	164; 104-289 (13)	122.9; 37-196 (38)	0.002
Random fasting urine						
Calcium/creat mmol/mmol	0.48; 0.28-0.99 (16)	0.33; 0.04-0.82 (33)	0.003	0.65; 0.18-0.76 (11)	0.31; 0.09-0.84 (40)	0.013
Citrate/creat mmol/mmol	0.20; 0.09-0.54 (16)	0.16; 0.06-0.49 (33)	0.062	0.31; 0.06-0.59 (12)	0.27; 0.04-0.67 (39)	0.617
$TmPO_4$/GFR mmol/l	0.78; 0.51-1.25 (14)	0.78; 0.50-1.68 (26)	0.755	0.94; 0.58-1.18 (12)	0.97; 0.48-1.53 (34)	0.491

† All ≥ 18 years of age, including family members and spouses, stone formers and non-stone formers. †† Mann-Whitney U-test P <0.05 statistically significant. Abbreviations as for Table 1.

Table 3. Comparison of data for all adults with $TmPO_4$ /GFR below 0.80 mmol/l (low) and ≥ 0.80 mmol/l[†]

	MEN TmPO4/GFR <0.80 mmol/l median; range (n)	MEN TmPO4/GFR ≥ 0.80 mmol/l median; range (n)	P[††] low v normal	WOMEN TmPO4/GFR <0.80 mmol/l median; range (n)	WOMEN TmPO4/GFR ≥ 0.80 mmol/l median; range (n)	P low v normal
Total in group[†††]	23	18		8	38	
stones	14 (61%)	9 (50%)	0.539	5 (63%)	9 (24%)	0.044
Age years	58; 27-89 (23)	43; 23-74 (18)	0.004	45; 29-60 (8)	41; 18-84 (38)	0.761
Plasma						
Bicarbonate mmol/l	28; 23-33 (23)	28; 22-32 (18)	0.426	26; 24-27 (8)	27; 21-31 (37)	0.027
Calcium mmol/l	2.40; 2.28-2.61 (23)	2.35; 2.24-2.52 (18)	0.151	2.34; 2.23-2.36 (8)	2.35; 2.20-2.59 (38)	0.151
Phosphate mmol/l	0.93; 0.71-1.10 (23)	1.17; 0.96-1.40 (18)	<0.001	0.85; 0.71-1.00 (8)	1.17; 0.87-1.40 (38)	<0.001
Urate mmol/l	0.32; 0.20-0.49 (23)	0.29; 0.22-0.48 (18)	0.252	0.30; 0.20-0.35 (8)	0.19; 0.09-0.41 (37)	0.008
Creatinine μmol/l	100; 76-101 (23)	87; 76-105 (18)	0.006	76; 54-82 (8)	74; 56-97 (38)	0.816
PTH pmol/l	4.0; 1.1-15.8 (23)	2.8; 1.3-5.9 (18)	0.009	3.6; 2.2-7.6 (8)	2.7; 0.6-8.1 (38)	0.164
1,25-DHCC pmol/l	108; 46-150 (22)	85; 52-159 (17)	0.497	97; 65-146 (8)	105; 38-180 (36)	0.670
24h urine						
Calcium mmol/24h	6.68; 1.38-16.81 (23)	6.36; 3.34-12.47 (17)	0.935	7.41; 2.99-18.58 (8)	3.67; 1.17-8.68 (38)	0.012
Citrate mmol/24h	3.01; 0.05-11.27 (23)	3.03; 0.70-8.49 (17)	0.935	3.93; 2.08-7.19 (8)	2.68; 0.35-5.74 (37)	0.030
Creatinine clearance l/24h	147; 36-263 (23)	164; 113-274 (17)	0.113	164; 101-289 (8)	134; 37-205 (38)	0.021
Volume l/24h	1.60: 0.78-2.64 (23)	1.59; 0.93-2.63 (17)	0.805	1.54; 0.66-3.44 (8)	1.52; 0.49-3.91 (38)	0.685
Fasting urine pH	5.95; 5.2-7.1 (20)	6.05; 5.0-8.3 (16)	0.610	5.60; 4.8-6.3 (7)	6.05; 5.0-7.2 (32)	0.056

[†] All ≥ 18 years of age, including family members and spouses, stone formers and non-stone formers.Two stone formers (one male, one female) and one female non-stone former with primary hyperparathyroidism have been excluded; [††] Mann-Whitney U-test , $P <0.05$ statistically significant. [†††]23/41 (56%) of the men and 8/46 (17%) of the women had TmPO4/GFR <0.80 mmol/l ($P< 0.001$). Abbreviations as for Table 1.

Association of Hypercalciuria with Other Intermediate Traits

Hyperoxaluria

Mild hyperoxaluria (median 0.61 mmol/24h, observed range 0.51-0.94 mmol/24h) was observed in 14% of samples and did not differ between stone formers and non-stone formers. However, the increases showed clustering with the hypercalciuric families (1, 2, 11 and 13) and 24h oxalate excretion was significantly higher in hypercalciuric than normocalciuric men (medians 0.46 and 0.33 mmol/24h respectively, P 0.002, Table 2).

Hypocitraturia

Only 15% of individuals had a low 24h urine citrate excretion and there was no difference between stone formers and non-stone formers. Contrary to expectation, values were significantly *higher* for hypercalciuric than normocalciuric men (median values 4.06 and 2.59 mmol/24h, P 0.018) but this was not the case for women (Table 2). Low fasting urine citrate/creatinine ratios were a common finding (29% of adults) with no difference between stone formers and non-stone formers, and were observed in five of 34 subjects (15%) <18 y of age. Twenty of the 47 low values in adults were from families 12 and 13 (with incidences of 41% and 36%, respectively). If these families are excluded, the incidence for the remaining families was 24%.

Phosphaturia

The maximum renal tubular reabsorption of phosphate ($TmPO_4$/GFR) is a practical means of assessing overall tubular capacity for tubular phosphate reabsorption which is independent of GFR. [24] Low values are indicative of phosphaturia. Low values for $TmPO_4$/GFR (<0.80 mmol/l) were observed in 41% of subjects and in 12 of the 14 families. In four families (3, 6, 7 and 8) low $TmPO_4$/GFR was the most frequent abnormality. The incidence was significantly higher in men than women (56 % versus 17% P <0.001). In both men and women $TmPO_4$/ GFR correlated significantly with plasma phosphate (men r 0.91, 95% confidence intervals CI 0.83, 0.95 n= 41 P<0.001; women r 0.83, CI 0.71, 0.91 n=46, P<0.001), in men with age (r -0.42 CI -0.65,-0.12 n= 41, P 0.006; Figure 1), and in women with plasma urate (r -0.35 CI –0.59,-0.05 n= 45, P 0.019). There was no significant correlation with 24h urine calcium (for men r 0.07, P 0.654; women r -0.25, P 0.098). Among men, $TmPO_4$/GFR <0.80 mmol/l had similar frequency among stone formers and non-stone formers. Men with values <0.80 mmol/l were older than those with a normal value and had higher plasma creatinine and PTH levels, perhaps a reflection of age. In contrast, compared with women with normal $TmPO_4/GFR$, more women with $TmPO_4/GFR$ <0.80 mmol/l were stone formers (63% versus 24%; P 0.044, Table 3), they had a small, but significant, reduction in plasma bicarbonate, increased plasma urate which was not associated with an increase in plasma creatinine, and significantly higher 24h calcium and citrate excretion and creatinine clearance. These increases were not explained by differences in 24h urine volume. It is feasible that these differences and phosphaturia were manifestations of a common underlying disturbance.

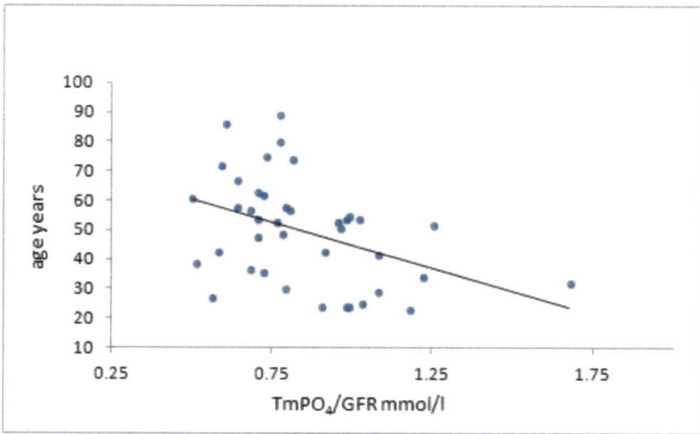

Figure 1. Correlation of TmPO4/GFR with age for all men ≥ 18 years of age in the family study. These included stone formers and non-stone formers, family members and spouses. Spearman's correlation coefficient r -0.42; 95% CI -0.65, -0.12 P 0.006.

Plasma 1,25-dihydroxycholecalciferol (1,25-DHCC)

We did not have our own reference data, and used the upper reference limit of 110 pmol/l provided with the assay kit. In view of the high frequency of raised values recorded (39%) this may have been too low. There was a similar incidence of raised values in men and women, and high values were not confined to the hypercalciuric families (Table 1). More men with raised values were stone formers than men with normal levels (68% versus 36%; P 0.039). A notable observation was that the 24h urine calcium excretion of both men and women with raised 1,25-DHCC was significantly higher than that of individuals with normal values (median calcium excretion for men 7.50 and 4.97 mmol/24h, P 0.004; for women 5.06 and 3.19 mmol/24h, P 0.014). This was not explained by differences in 24h urine volume: for men, the median volumes were 1.61 and 1.60 l/24h, P 0.679, and for women with raised 1,25-DHCC, 1.49 versus 1.60 l/24h, P 0.429. Fasting urine calcium/creatinine ratios were also higher but not significantly different (median values for men 0.42 and 0.32 mmol/mmol, P 0.070; for women 0.40 and 0.30 mmol/mmol, P 0.077). There were no differences in age, plasma phosphate, creatinine, creatinine clearance, PTH or $TmPO_4$/GFR. The combined data for stone forming and non-stone forming men showed significant correlation between 1,25-DHCC and 24h urine calcium excretion : r 0.56, CI 0.30, 0.74 n=44, P<0.001, and fasting calcium/creatinine ratio: r 0.44, CI 0.16, 0.65 n=46, P 0.002. For women, there was significant correlation with 24h urine calcium: r 0.41, CI 0.14, 0.62, P 0.004, but not with calcium/creatinine ratio (P 0.101). There was no significant correlation in men or women between 1,25-DHCC and plasma calcium, phosphate, PTH or $TmPO_4$/GFR and hence there was no apparent explanation for increased 1,25-DHCC levels.

Plasma PTH

PTH was increased in only 8 individuals (8% of those tested) and was therefore a relatively uncommon finding. In three of the subjects, the biochemical findings were consistent with primary hyperparathyroidism. In two others who were normocalcemic and elderly (86y and 80y) the increases may have been attributable to ageing.

DNA Microsatellite Linkage Analyses

None of the LOD scores for linkage of any of the six microsatellite markers with stone formation, hypercalciuria or phosphaturia were indicative of linkage disequilibrium. This is strong, although not conclusive, evidence that in these pedigrees the genes for the CASR, SLC34A1, vitamin D receptor and NPT2 are not susceptibility loci for these abnormalities.

However, an analysis of the individual quantitative traits among all sib pairs in the study identified a possible link between fasting urinary citrate/creatinine ratio and the D5S614 marker for the *NPT2* gene with a summated LOD score of 2.54. There was also a weak positive signal with 24-hour urinary citrate and D5S614. When the analysis of linkage was restricted to the two hypocitraturic families a LOD score of 4.99 was obtained for linkage between fasting urinary citrate/creatinine ratio and D5S614. This link was supported by a weak positive signal between fasting urinary citrate/creatinine ratio and D5S1354 (LOD score 0.6). Retrospectively, it was then possible to show that all the evidence for linkage between D5S614 and fasting citrate/creatinine ratio arose from a single family (Family 12) with a LOD score of 6.56. Subsequently, we demonstrated that four other microsatellite markers located close to the *NPT2* gene were also in linkage disequilibrium with a locus controlling fasting urinary citrate/creatinine ratio in this family. A mutation scan of the *NPT2* gene would have been the logical next step to look for an abnormality and, if confirmed, functional studies of the cloned gene. Unfortunately these investigations were not readily available at the time of the study.

Overview of the Observations for Hypercalciuria

The findings from this small study confirm that hypercalciuria is a familial abnormality in some, but not all, stone-forming kindreds, that it increases the risk for stones, and is sometimes associated with hyperoxaluria which may also be familial and, of some surprise, in men with increased urinary citrate which is believed to protect against calcium stones. From a large epidemiological study Curhan also reported, as a new and inexplicable observation, that 24h urine citrate was increased in male stone formers with a family history of stones. [18] In our families, there was no demonstrable linkage of hypercalciuria with the genes for the CASR, SLC34A1, vitamin D receptor and NPT2. Phosphaturia, as evidenced by low $TmPO_4/GFR$ values, was common, but was a non-specific abnormality since the frequency was similar among normocalciuric individuals. $TmPO_4/GFR$ decreased with age in men. There was no demonstrable linkage of low $TmPO_4/GFR$ with the *NPT2* phosphate transporter gene. Plasma 1,25-DHCC was higher in hypercalciuric than normocalciuric subjects. This increase could not be attributed to differences in PTH or plasma phosphate.

Studies from the Stone Clinic Database

We have recently analyzed the data for stone formers investigated in the clinic from 1990 to July 2007, and now summarize the published findings from three of the investigations. [21-23] There were clearly sex differences for many parameters, particularly those related to creatinine, and we have analyzed the data for men and women separately in all of our studies.

Study 1: An Overview of the Data for the Full Clinic Cohort

We reviewed the data for the full patient cohort of 816 women and 1983 men (ratio 1:2.43). [21] Important observations were differences in the frequencies of stone risk factors between men and women, and changes with age. Relevant results are summarized in Table 4. They confirm the high familial incidence of stones and showed a significantly higher frequency of women with a first degree affected relative (24%) than men (19%). Overall, the observations are similar to those reported from other large clinics. As is well-recognized, [2, 4, 8, 25] hypercalciuria, hyperoxaluria and hyperuricosuria were more common in men. Excretion of calcium, oxalate and urate were significantly correlated. The frequency of hypocitraturia was high using our lower reference limit of 1.60 mmol/24h, derived in-house from healthy volunteers. Bias in patient selection may be partly responsible since 24h urine citrate was not measured routinely, but more often in recurrent stone formers or patients with underlying clinical disorders associated with hypocitraturia. Applying diagnostic thresholds of 2.0 and 1.7 mmol/24h, two studies reported hypocitraturia in 30% and 32.7% of recurrent stone formers. [8, 26] One large study found no difference in citrate excretion between stone formers and controls. [27] These observations make the finding of *raised* urinary citrate levels in hypercalciuric subjects in our family study even more surprising. Low values for $TmPO_4$/GFR, found frequently among our patients, are discussed below.

We compared the data for hypercalciuric and normocalciuric patients with no evident underlying clinical disorder to cause stones ('idiopathic' stone formers). Table 5 presents indices which were significantly different. Hypercalciuria was associated with higher excretion of oxalate and urate, but also with small increases in the 24h urinary volume. Errors in timing of the 24h collections might have over-estimated the calculated 24h oxalate and urate excretion. However, these were large patient groups and there is no reason why hypercalciuric individuals should have made mistakes more often than normocalciuric patients. The calcium *concentration* of their urine was significantly higher. Age, plasma calcium, phosphate, PTH, and $TmPO_4$/GFR did not differ significantly.

Table 4. Overview of relevant data from the stone clinic data base

Variable Median; 2.5-97.5 percentiles	Women	no.	Men	no.	Women & men compared P
Final cohort: n=2799	816 (29%)		1983 (71%)		1:2.43
Age (years)	49; 20-79	811	49; 23-77	1968	
Age at first stone episode (years)	44; 28-75	805	43;28-73	1968	
Recurrent stones	184 (23%)		663 (33%)		<0.001
No. (%) with first degree relatives with stones					
one relative	153 (19%)		314 (16%)		
two relatives	26 (3%)		49 (3%)		
three or more relatives	14 (2%)		10 (<1%)		
total	193 (24%)		373 (19%)		0.004
Plasma Creatinine (µmol/l) *Ref :women 53-97µmol/l* *men 80-115µmol/l*	77; 56-116	760	93; 72-129	1787	<0.001
Phosphate: mmol/l *Ref 0.70-1.50 mmol/l*	1.02; 0.68-1.34	778	0.92; 0.60-1.29	1889	<0.001
$TmPO_4$/GFR: mmol/l *Ref: 0.80-1.35 mmol/l*	0.91; 0.54-1.48	563	0.82; 0.46-1.35	1380	<0.001
No. <0.80 mmol/l	165 (29%)		638 (46%)		<0.001
No. <0.70 mmol/l	73 (13%)		341 (25%)		<0.001
24h urine †	n=597		n= 1490		
Calcium: mmol/24h Ref: women 2.00-6.25mmol/24h men 2.00-7.50 mmol/24h	5.20; 1.62-12.27	593	7.10; 2.35-14.59	1486	<0.001
no. above ref range	186 (31%)		646 (43%)		<0.001

Table 4. (Continued)

Variable Median; 2.5-97.5 percentiles no.	Women		Men		Women & men compared P
Oxalate: mmol/24h *Ref: < 0.50 mmol/24h*	0.32; 0.18-0.65	564	0.40; 0.21-0.73	1423	<0.001
no. above ref range	38 (7%)		239 (17%)		<0.001
Uric acid: mmol/24h *Ref: women < 4.50 mmol/24h* *men < 4.80 mmol/24h*	3.18;1.64-6.27	222	3.93; 2.01-6.90	708	<0.001
no. above ref range	23 (10%)		159 (22%)		<0.001
Citrate: mmol/24h *Ref: 1.52- 7.00 mmol/24h*	1.73; 0.29-6.25	152	1.62; 0.38-4.58	372	0.051
no. below ref range	64 (42%)		172 (46%)		0.439
Creatinine: mmol/24h *ref: men ≥10.60 mmol/24h* *women ≥7.00 mmol/24h*	10.00; 7.20-15.41	597	15.30; 10.90-22.00	1490	<0.001
Creatinine clearance: l/24h *ref: men 135-200 l/24h* *women 120-180 l/24h*	134.0; 70.2-223.8	528	165.0; 98.0-242.0	1267	<0.001

† After excluding samples with low 24h urine creatinine and hence probably incomplete collections (men <10.60 mmol/24h, n= 175 ; women <7.00 mmol/24h, n= 80) and with no recorded 24h urine creatinine (men 318; women 139); $TmPO_4/GFR$= renal threshold of phosphate concentration. Statistically significant differences between men and women: $P<0.05$, Mann-Whitney U test for continuous variables; Chi square with Yate's correction or Fisher's exact test for contingency comparisons. Adapted from Walker et al. Ann Clin Biochem 2013;50: 127-39 [21] Reproduced with permission from Sage Publications Ltd.

Table 5. Comparison of data for idiopathic stone formers with hypercalciuria and normocalciuria

	MEN urine calcium > 7.50 mmol/24h Median; range[†] (n)	MEN urine calcium ≤ 7.50 mmol/24h Median; range (n)	P[††] high v normal	WOMEN urine calcium > 6.25 mmol/24h Median; range (n)	WOMEN urine calcium ≤ 6.25 mmol/24h Median; range (n)	P high v normal
Total in group[†††]	276	347		133	278	
Age with first stone years	41; 10-79 (276)	43; 9-78 (347)	0.035	42; 10-76 (131)	42; 9-94 (276)	0.661
Age at the clinic years	46; 20-80 (276)	48; 19-92 (347)	0.070	45; 18-76 (131)	45; 15-94 (276)	0.761
Plasma						
Calcium mmol/l	2.37; 2.13-2.54 (276)	2.37; 2.14-2.55 (347)	0.526	2.35; 2.14-2.53 (133)	2.36; 2.11-2.59 (278)	0.237
Phosphate mmol/l	0.93; 0.34-1.34 (270)	0.93; 0.52-1.46 (335)	0.747	1.00; 0.66-1.36 (128)	1.03; 0.60-1.63 (270)	0.179
PTH[††††] pmol/l	2.9; 1.0-7.3 (208)	3.0; 1.0-7.2 (267)	0.240	2.9; 1.2-7.3 (99)	3.3; 0.7-7.3 (195)	0.539
24h urine						
Calcium mmol/24h >10.00mmol/24h	9.30;7.56-19.40 (276) 101 (36%)	5.80; 2.21-7.50 (347)	<0.001	7.80; 6.30-18.60 (133) 17 (13%)	4.60; 2.00-6.24 (278)	<0.001
Calcium mmol/l	9.30;1.80-13.30 (276)	5.80;0.67-9.36 (347)	<0.001	7.80;1.50-13.86 (133)	4.60;0.70-11.29 (278)	<0.001
Oxalate mmol/24h >0.50 mmol/24h	0.41; 0.09-0.87 (272) 45 (17%)	0.38; 0.13-1.45 (338) 40 (12%)	<0.001	0.32; 0.12-0.90 (123) 11 (8%)	0.31; 0.08-1.29 (265) 12 (5%)	0.002
Urate mmol /24h Increased: m > 4.8; f >4.5 mmol/24h	3.99;1.22-10.18 (114) 28 (25%)	3.78; 1.86-8.40 (145) 23 (16%)	0.048	3.52; 1.41-7.80 (37) 8 (16%)	3.10; 1.54-7.00 (102) 8 (8%)	0.058
Citrate mmol/24h <1.60 mmol/24h	1.88; 0.44-6.00 (66) 25 (38%)	1.66; 0.36-4.95 (75) 35 (47%)	0.315	1.97; 0.68-7.00 (30) 12 (40%)	2.18; 0.30-6.98 (70) 26 (37%)	0.925
urine volume l/24h	1.95; 0.73-5.23 (272)	1.73; 0.63-5.08 (344)	<0.001	1.84; 0.76-4.75 (130)	1.69; 0.48-4.17 (278)	0.043

Table 5. (Continued)

	MEN urine calcium > 7.50 mmol/24h Median; range[†] (n)	**MEN** urine calcium ≤ 7.50 mmol/24h Median; range (n)	P[††] high v normal	**WOMEN** urine calcium > 6.25 mmol/24h Median; range (n)	**WOMEN** urine calcium ≤ 6.25 mmol/24h Median; range (n)	P high v normal
Random urine						
pH	6.20; 4.30-7.78 (258)	6.10; 4.50-8.00 (337)	0.045	6.04; 4.85-7.70 (124)	6.00; 4.50-8.00 (261)	0.990
$TmPO_4$/GFR mmol/l <0.80 mmol/l <0.70 mmol/l	0.82; 0.24-1.60 (198) 87 (44%) 43 (22%)	0.86; 0.29-1.99 (256) 99 (39%) 48 (19%)	0.112	0.91; 0.54-1.82 (88) 26 (30%) 13 (15%)	0.92; 0.25-2.12 (188) 45 (24%) 13 (7%)	0.527

[†] Median and observed ranges; [††] Mann-Whitney U-test; P <0.05 statistically significant.
[†††] 276/ 623 (44%) men & 133/411 (32%) of the women had hypercalciuria (P <0.001); [††††] Three PTH assay kits were used; only the results for the first kit used to 2001 are shown.

Table 6. Comparison of data for hypercalciuric male stone formers with filtered calcium in the lowest and highest quintiles (n = 55 per quintile)

	Lowest quintile median; 2.5-97.5 percentiles	**no. of observations**	**Highest quintile median; 2.5-97.5 percentiles**	**no. of observations**	**Lowest v highest quintile p**
Age of first stone (years)	44; 19-71	55	37; 19-60	55	0.012
Age at clinic (years)	52; 29-75	55	40; 24-60	55	<0.001
Positive family history	11 (20%)	55	15 (27%)	55	0.501
Recurrent stones	22 (40%)	55	19 (35%)	55	0.694
Plasma					
Ultrafiltrable calcium (mmol/l) ref 1.29-1.53	1.41; 1.30-1.49	55	1.43; 1.33-1.50	55	0.007

	Lowest quintile median; 2.5-97.5 percentiles	no. of observations	Highest quintile median; 2.5-97.5 percentiles	no. of observations	Lowest v highest quintile p
PTH † (pmol/l) ref <7.3	2.9; 1.3-6.7	40	2.8; 1.4-5.0	43	0.553
Urine					
Calcium (mmol/24h) ref 2.00-7.50	8.70; 7.67-12.50	55	10.50; 7.77-18.58	55	<0.001
Filtered calcium (mmol/24h)	194.8; 140.2-211.1	55	318.1; 296.0-366.4	55	<0.001
Reabsorbed calcium (mmol/24h)	184.5; 131.2-202.2	55	307.7; 285.2-357.0	55	<0.001
Oxalate (mmol/24h) ref <0.50	0.35; 0.17-0.53	54	0.45; 0.32-0.75	54	<0.001
Urate (mmol/24h) ref <4.80	3.41; 2.23-6.00	26	4.73; 3.51-6.89	20	<0.001
Creatinine (mmol/24h)	13.20; 10.87-18.16	55	19.70; 15.44-23.29	55	<0.001
Creatinine clearance (l/24h)	140.0; 96.7-154.7	55	224.1; 201.5-253.3	55	<0.001
Volume (l/24h)	2.03; 0.85-4.44	55	1.81; 1.06-3.60	55	0.490
pH	6.25; 5.13-7.44	54	6.07; 5.10-7.55	52	0.656
$TmPO_4$/GFR (mmol/l) ref 0.80-1.35	0.85; 0.60-1.14	43	0.83; 0.60-1.29	41	0.816
Stone composition	**n = 30**		**n = 25**		
calcium oxalate	4 (13%)		5 (20%)		0.717
calcium oxalate phosphate	24 (80%)		17 (68%)		0.363

PTH parathyroid hormone; † three assay kits for PTH were used with differing sensitivities; only the results obtained up to December 2001 using the first assay kit are shown. Statistical comparisons: Mann-Whitney U test for continuous variables; Fisher's exact test for contingency comparisons; $P < 0.05$ statistically significant. Adapted from Walker et al: J Clin Pathol 2014; 67(4): 355-360.[22] Reproduced with permission from BMJ Publishing Group Ltd.

Table 7. Data for hyperuricosuric male stone formers: all 30 with filtered urate below the median for normouricosuria ('low filtered urate') compared with the 30 with the highest filtration ('high filtered urate')

	Hyperuricosuria[†] Low filtered urate median; 2.5-97.5 percentiles	n	Hyperuricosuria High filtered urate median; 2.5-97.5 percentiles	n	Low v. high filtered urate P
Age of first stone years	37; 15-69	30	41; 16-61	29	0.617
Age at clinic years	45; 27-70	30	47; 26-62	30	0.469
First degree relative	6 (20%)	30	2 (7%)	30	0.254
Recurrent stones	14 (47%)	30	13 (43%)	30	1.000
eGFR ml/min/m^2	80; 51-110	30	85; 62-123	30	0.141
Plasma					
Urate mmol/l	0.29; 0.17-0.43	30	0.46; 0.37-0.59	30	<0.001
Calcium mmol/l	2.35; 2.22-2.57	30	2.39; 2.30-2.51	29	0.097
Creatinine μmol/l	96; 74-136	30	91; 70-116	30	0.169
Biochemical risk factors					
Urine urate mmol/24h	5.60; 4.89-8.53	30	5.84; 4.90-8.29	30	0.171
Filtered urate mmol/24h	47.4; 29.3-51.6	30	96.7; 85.2-115.7	30	<0.001
Percentage of urate reabsorbed	87.0; 74.5-90.3	30	93.6; 91.7-95.6	30	<0.001
Urine oxalate mmol/24h Urine oxalate >0.50 mmol/24h	0.42; 0.23-0.94 7 (25%)	28	0.53; 0.31-0.71 15(56%)	27	0.014 0.029
Urine calcium mmol/24h Urine calcium >7.50 mmol/24h	8.17; 4.45-15.54 20 (67%)	30	7.79; 3.29-16.51 15 (50%)	30	0.554 0.295
Urine volume l/24h	1.84; 0.71-3.50	30	1.80; 1.24-3.85	30	0.965
Random urine pH	5.99; 5.00-7.52	28	5.64; 4.92-7.17	28	0.206
$TmPO_4$/GFR mmol/l[††] <0.70 mmol/L	0.78; 0.50-1.00 8 (40%)	20	0.94; 0.64-1.21 4 (22%)	18	0.019 0.307
Creatinine clearance l/24h >200 l/24h	154.5; 112.2-225.5 5 (17%)	30	219.5; 157.3-266.6 22 (73%)	30	<0.001 <0.001

[†] Hyperuricosuria: urinary urate >4.80 mmol/24h; [††] $TmPO_4$/GFR renal threshold of phosphate concentration; Statistical comparisons: Mann-Whitney U test for continuous variables; Fisher's exact test for contingency comparisons; $P < 0.05$ statistically significant. Adapted from Walker et al., Urolithiasis 2014; 42 (4) 291-300 [23]. Reproduced with kind permission from Springer Science + Business Media.

Phosphaturia

Our clinic is unusual in that we estimate $TmPO_4$ /GFR. This investigation is seldom included in front-line clinic screening protocols for stone risk factors. After excluding patients with abnormal PTH concentrations, $TmPO_4$/GFR of 44% of men and of 24% of women was below a reference limit of 0.80mmol/l [24] ($P<0.001$), and of 22% of men and 8% of women was < 0.70mmol/l ($P <0.001$). The incidence was no higher in hypercalciuric than normocalciuric stone formers, which is in keeping with the lack of an association with hypercalciuria observed in our family study. Rendina *et al.* identified a sub-set of stone formers with evidence of a renal phosphate leak on the basis of fasting levels of plasma phosphate below the reference range, $TmPO_4$/GFR <0.70 mmol/l and a normal plasma PTH concentration. [28] In our cohort, 6% of men and 1.6% of women had similar biochemical abnormalities and probably fell within this category, although the samples were usually non-fasting. Compared with stone formers with normal PTH, plasma phosphate and $TmPO_4$/GFR >0.80 mmol/l, the men with a phosphate leak were older and had higher plasma creatinine and lower plasma calcium concentrations (2.35; 2.20-2.50 mmol/l, n = 72; controls 2.38; 2.22-2.54 mmol/l, n = 618; P = 0.001). In a similar comparison for women, the seven with a phosphate leak had lower plasma bicarbonate concentrations (median 25 range 23-28 mmol/l, n = 7; controls 28, range 23-34 mmol/l, n = 303; P = 0.001), and more often had a first degree relative with stones (71% versus 28% P = 0.008). There were no other significant differences. It is interesting that in our family study, women with low TmPO4/GFR also had a small decrease in plasma bicarbonate.

Data for phosphaturia among stone formers are sparse. [8] Phosphaturia cannot be diagnosed from measurement of 24h urine phosphate, unless this is undertaken during metabolic balance studies, since this largely reflects dietary phosphate intake. One study reported lower $TmPO_4$/GFR in calcium stone formers with normal PTH compared with normal subjects, [29] and another found evidence of a phosphate leak (see above) in 20% of stone formers. [28] The explanation for the high frequency of phosphaturia found in stone patients is unknown. In our clinic, collection of non-fasting samples may have inflated the incidence. Among patients with low $TmPO_4$/GFR values, Prié *et al.* identified two with mutations of the gene for NPT2a, one with renal stones and the other with osteoporosis, and in seven other phosphaturic patients, found mutations of the *NHERF-1* gene (see below). [30, 31] Activity of NPT2a is controlled by PTH, by pH (activity is decreased at low pH) and by fibroblast growth factor-23 (FGF23). FGF23 is a phosphaturic hormone produced in bone which binds to the apical membrane of the proximal tubules with a renally-produced protein, klotho, and suppresses NPT2 activity. [32] Rare mutations of the *FGF23* gene cause phosphaturia, [32] but we are not aware of any reports linking gene polymorphisms with stones. A polymorphism of the klotho gene has been associated with an increased risk for renal stones. [33] *NPT2a* and *NHERF-1* mutations appear to occur too rarely to explain the high frequency of phosphaturia in stone formers, and it seems more likely that this abnormality is a response to some other biochemical disturbance, possibly of H^+ secretion.

Study 2: Investigation of Male Clinic Patients with Idiopathic Hypercalciuria [22]

In this data base study, our first objective was to segregate male stone formers with idiopathic hypercalciuria due to impaired renal tubular handling of calcium (renal hypercalciuria) from those filtering increased amounts of calcium into the kidneys. This distinction will be fundamental for future meaningful genetic studies. Our second aim was to find out whether associated risk factors for stone production differed between these two groups of men.

Study 2 (a) Identification of Male Stone Formers with Renal Hypercalciuria

Because we wanted to minimize the effects of variations in plasma calcium levels on the amount of calcium delivered to the kidney, we selected men from the data base who had normal levels of plasma ultrafiltrable calcium, which we estimated as 60% of total plasma calcium adjusted for albumin. We obtained this figure from reported observations in experimental animals, and healthy adult volunteers and stone formers. [11, 34, 35] Measurement of ultrafiltrable calcium of large numbers of clinic patients is not feasible, and measurement of ionized calcium excludes complexed calcium. With normal plasma PTH and bicarbonate levels and good renal function errors will be very small.

Men were included if they had idiopathic calcium stones, no disorder or drug treatment associated with abnormalities of ionized plasma calcium or calcium excretion, did not have diabetes mellitus or gout, had two well-functioning kidneys with normal plasma creatinine and bicarbonate, estimated GFR (eGFR) $\geq$ 60 ml/ min/ 1.73 m^2 and no structural abnormality of the urinary tract, if their 24h urine sample was probably complete (creatinine $\geq$

10.60 mmol/24h), [27] and urine calcium was >2.00 mmol/24h. We estimated the amount of calcium filtered daily as ultrafiltrable plasma calcium x creatinine clearance, which we used as an approximation for glomerular filtration rate (GFR). The amount of calcium reabsorbed per 24h was the difference between filtered calcium and 24h urine calcium. The final study cohort of 623 men comprised 276 (44%) with hypercalciuria and 347 with normocalciuria. They had similar plasma concentrations of ultrafiltrable calcium (P 0.598). At each level of filtered calcium there was wide inter-individual variation in the percentage of filtered calcium which was reabsorbed (Figure 2). As predicted from the calculation, for any given amount of filtered calcium, hypercalciuric men reabsorbed less calcium than normocalciuric men—a new observation for a clinic population, which is only demonstrable by relating filtered calcium to excreted calcium. This observation implies that reduced renal tubular reabsorption is a common abnormality in idiopathic hypercalciuria. Others have found that renal calcium reabsorption is reduced in small groups of carefully selected stone formers with idiopathic hypercalciuria [7, 11, 36, 37] Ninety three (34%) of the hypercalciuric men had values for filtered calcium below the median for men with normocalciuria. It was inferred that reduced reabsorption of filtered calcium was the dominant abnormality in these men.

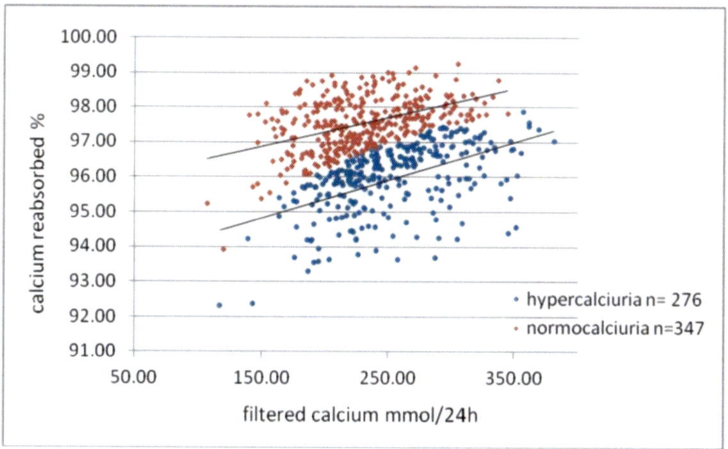

Figure 2. Correlation between filtered calcium and percentage reabsorbed by 623 male stone formers with idiopathic calcium stones. Spearman's coefficient r (95% CI): for hypercalciuric men: r 0.56, CI 0.47, 0.52, P <0.001; for normocalciuric men r 0.43, CI 0.34, 0.52, P < 0.001. Walker et al. 2014, J Clin Pathol 67 (4): 355-360[22]. Figure reproduced with permission from BMJ Publishing Group Ltd.

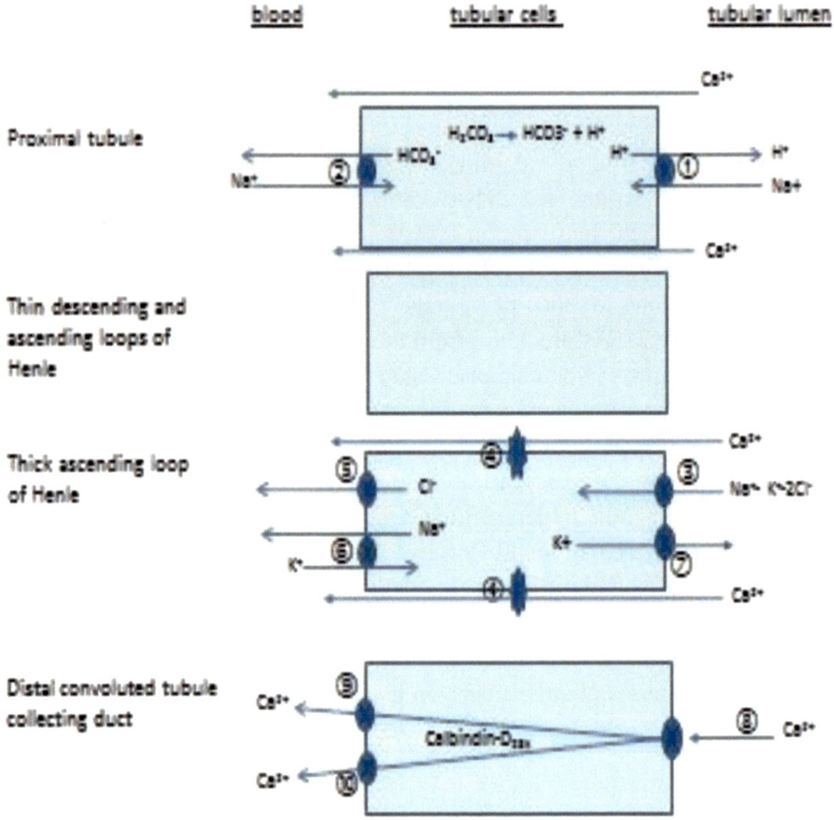

Figure 3. Reabsorption of filtered calcium by the renal tubules. Approximately 65% is reabsorbed in the proximal tubule by the paracellular route, none in the thin descending and ascending loops of Henle, around 25% by the paracellular route in the thick ascending loop of Henle, and 8-10% by trans-cellular transport in the distal nephron. Key:
1 NHE3 (Na^{+}/H^{+} antiporter)*
2 NBCe1 ($HCO3^{-}$ Na^{+} exchanger)*
3 NKCC2 (NA-K-Cl cotransporter 2)*
4 Claudin-16 (paracellin-1)
5 Chloride channel CLC-Kb
6 Na^{+}-K^{+}-ATPase
7 ROMK (ATP-sensitive inwardly rectifying K channel)
8 TRPV5 (transient receptor potential vanilloid member 5 protein)
9 PMCA (plasma membrane Ca^{2+} ATPase)
10 NCX (Na^{+} / Ca^{2+} exchanger)
* These transporters are also involved in H^{+} secretion and NH_3 buffering

Study 2 (b) Comparison of Stone Risk Factors of Men with Hypercalciuria due to Reduced Renal Reabsorption of Calcium and Those with a High Filtered Load

We then compared stone risk factors of the 55 hypercalciuric men in the lowest filtration quintile with the 55 in the highest (Table 6). The recurrence rate for stones and incidence of a first degree relative with stones were high, and similar, in both groups. The men with high calcium filtration reabsorbed a very large proportion of the filtered load but not enough to achieve a normal 24h urinary calcium excretion. Compared with men in the lowest quintile, they had higher 24h urine calcium, oxalate and urate excretion and, of greater significance for stone risk, higher urinary concentrations per liter of calcium, oxalate and urate. These increases could account for their younger age at their first stone episode and at the time of referral to the clinic. The incidence of phosphaturia was similar and high in both groups, and plasma PTH and urine pH were not significantly different.

Mechanism of Decreased Renal Reabsorption of Calcium

Genetic variation in the renal handling of calcium seems the most likely explanation for decreased calcium reabsorption in hypercalciuria. Because of the stringent selection criteria for this study, other possible causes [38, 39] were considered to be highly unlikely, although we cannot exclude a high dietary sodium consumption [8, 39] since urinary sodium excretion was not recorded on the database. A familial risk for stones has been well documented. [4, 7, 15, 18, 19] One study reported a frequency of 16.8% of a first degree affected relative of men and 22.7% of women with stones compared with 6% of controls. [40] There was a high incidence of patients with first degree relatives with stones in our cohort, and heritability was clearly evident in our family study. Our findings in the family study strongly support inheritance of hypercalciuria.

Calcium Reabsorption by the Renal Tubules

Reabsorption of calcium by the renal tubules is now known to occur through the highly co-ordinated activities of a growing number of identified renal transport processes. [4, 12, 13, 15, 41] Others will almost certainly be discovered. Calcium reabsorption is closely integrated with the transport of H^+ ions, phosphate and other anions and some transporters are structurally associated through binding to common intracellular scaffolding proteins. [42, 43] Figure 3 presents a simplified overview. Briefly, circulating ionized and complexed calcium is filtered into the kidneys and normally around 98% is subsequently reabsorbed back into the blood. Most (around 65%) is reabsorbed in the proximal tubules, none in the thin ascending and descending loops of Henle, around 25% in the thick ascending limb of loop of Henle (TAL) and 8-10% in the distal convoluted tubule and collecting duct. It is in the distal nephron that calcium reabsorption is finely controlled by PTH and 1,25-DHCC. Calcium sensing receptors (CASR), located on the apical membranes of the cells lining the proximal tubules and inner medullary collecting duct, and the basolateral membranes of cells in the TAL and the distal nephron, monitor luminal and blood calcium levels and regulate calcium reabsorption. In the proximal tubule most calcium is reabsorbed by the paracellular route driven by the lumen positive potential difference generated by the Na^+/H^+ antiporter NHE3 which is the principal sodium proximal tubular transporter. Absorption from the TAL similarly is paracellular, in this case driven by a lumen positive voltage generated by the bumetamide-sensitive Na^+-K^+-Cl^- cotransporter (NKCC2). Intracellular Na^+ and Cl^- concentrations are maintained by the activities of Na^+/K^+-ATPase and the chloride channel CLC-Kb. K^+ is transported back into the tubular lumen by the ATP-sensitive inwardly rectifying potassium (ROMK) channel creating the voltage which drives Ca^{2+} into the blood through claudin-16 (paracellin -1) tight junctions. In the distal nephron calcium is actively reabsorbed. It enters the cells by the transient receptor potential vanilloid member 5 protein (TRPV5) channel, is transported through the cells bound to calbindin-D_{28k} and exported via the Na^+/Ca^{2+} exchanger (NCX) and plasma membrane Ca^{2+} ATPase (PMCA). [12, 44]

Genetic Abnormalities which Cause Hypercalciuria

Hypercalciuria, nephrocalcinosis and nephrolithiasis are features of some inherited monogenic disorders, [4, 12, 13, 15, 41] but these are exceptionally rare and not likely to be encountered in a stone clinic. However, common polymorphisms of these and other so far unidentified genes which have a small variable effect on transporter function probably account for the inherited variation in calcium excretion in the general population. The profile of activities of the 'package' of transporter genes inherited will determine the susceptibility to hypercalciuria perhaps through a threshold effect. Co-inheritance of genes with polymorphisms associated with excretion of other stone risk factors, for example phosphate, oxalate or urate, will add to the genetic risk for stone formation. The search for polymorphisms of familiar renal calcium transporters has been unproductive so far. Two studies found a potential susceptibility locus near the vitamin D receptor gene but others found no evidence of linkage. An Italian study found a gain of function polymorphism of the CASR gene in women which was associated with an increased risk of hypercalciuria, but other studies reported negative findings, and others found no evidence of an association with the 1α-cholecalciferol hydroxylase gene. [4, 12, 13, 15, 41] In one large kindred there was linkage of absorptive hypercalciuria with the soluble adenyl cyclase gene, but the mechanism by which an abnormality of this enzyme would increase calcium excretion is unknown. [45] In our family study, we found no evidence of linkage of the genes for the CASR, thiazide-sensitive sodium chloride cotransporter, vitamin D receptor and NPT2 sodium-phosphate cotransporter-2 with hypercalciuria or phosphaturia. The linkage of NPT2 to fasting hypocitraturia in one kindred, indicates possible interaction of this pH dependent gene with renal citrate metabolism, which may be via H^+ secretion. An exciting fairly recent development has been the discovery of NHERF-1 and NHERF-2 which are members of a protein family called the Sodium-Hydrogen-Exchanger Regulatory Factor. They contain tandem domains (PDZ domains) which are recognized by a range of proteins. In rat and mouse kidney, NHERF-1 is highly expressed in the renal proximal tubule. It binds to a range of proteins which include NHE3, NPT2, the sodium-bicarbonate transporter and the PTH receptor. Binding with NHERF-1 targets NPT2 to the apical membrane and is essential for its activity, inhibits NHE3 and initiates degradation of the PTH receptor. NHERF-1 is estrogen-inducible. NHERF-1 knock-out mice have phosphaturia, hypercalciuria, hyperuricosuria, raised 1,25-DHCC and a tendency to low PTH. NHERF-2 is localized principally in the distal nephron and binds to TRPV5, the outer medullary potassium channel and H^+-ATPase. [42, 46-48] In our family study, hypercalciuria was significantly associated with raised 1,25-DHCC levels which could not be explained by hypophosphatemia or increases in plasma PTH and which might be consistent with an abnormality of NHERF-1.

Mechanisms Causing Hyperfiltration of Calcium

Higher calcium filtration of men in the top quintile was explained largely by their higher creatinine clearance which was above an upper reference limit of 200l/24h in 54 (98%) of cases. Inaccurately timed collections might have accounted for this, [49] but was an unlikely explanation for the group as a whole. [22]

Raised creatinine clearance was observed in one other study of hypercalciuric male recurrent stone formers on a free choice diet. Compared with normocalciuric recurrent stone formers and controls, they had increased renal mass and 24h urinary creatinine excretion and a higher ratio of plasma 1,25-DHCC to PTH which is an index of regulation of 1,25-DHCC production. [50] In another study of stone formers with idiopathic hypercalciuria, creatinine clearance decreased after 15 days of dietary protein restriction, but not significantly. There was a significant decrease in the ratio of plasma 1,25-DHCC to PTH. [51] There is a large body of evidence to show that high intakes of protein and amino acids increase GFR in animals and humans, whether this is measured by creatinine clearance or by other techniques which avoid interference from dietary creatine. [52-57] In short-term studies of healthy humans (≤ 3 weeks) the increase in GFR ranged from negligible to 20%. The increase was greater on diets maintained for months or years. [57] Acute protein loading causes a rapid increase in GFR which, in one study, reached a peak by 2.5h. [54] This has been associated with changes in intra-renal perfusion, [55] and in animal models, high protein feeding causes parallel changes in GFR and renal plasma flow indicating a hemodynamic response. In rats, renal size increases due to enlargement of both the renal tubules and glomeruli. [57] Despite extensive investigation, the mechanisms which cause the changes in intra-renal blood flow are still unclear. It has been proposed that increased production of the vasodilator nitric oxide (NO) from L-arginine in the kidneys may be responsible. [56, 57] Infusion of L-arginine or amino acid mixtures into isolated perfused kidneys increases renal blood flow, [57] and administration of an inhibitor of NO synthesis, N^G-monomethyl-L-arginine, via the renal artery into rats infused with amino acids significantly reduced the GFR and renal plasma flow. The NO hypothesis is attractive in view of our increased understanding of the processes which link dietary protein ingestion with renal NO synthesis. [58] In the kidneys, NO is produced by the arginine-citrulline–nitric oxide cycle. [59] The arginine substrate for this cycle derives mainly from citrulline which is synthesized in the small intestine from ingested amino acids and from endogenously produced glutamine. Endogenous glutamine production is increased after protein ingestion. Citrulline is transported from the intestine to the kidneys where it is converted to arginine and exported to the circulation or metabolized via the arginine-citrulline–nitric oxide cycle. High protein consumption could account for the high creatinine clearance values observed in our study through a true increase in GFR, exaggerated by a spurious increase due to a high creative intake from meat, [49] and hemodynamic changes within the kidney might have reduced the renal reabsorption of calcium. There is now a large body of evidence that high protein consumption increases urinary calcium excretion, [51, 60, and 61] and reduced renal absorption may be a contributory factor. However, this is speculative since, although discussed with the patients, protein intakes were not calculated. Dietary excesses together with increased GFR might also explain the higher oxalate and urate excretion in this group. [3, 8, 50] These abnormalities are frequently associated with a high protein intake. [51] Dietary protein restriction for 15 days led to significant decreases in urinary excretion of calcium, urate and oxalate. [51]

Study 3. Comparison of Risk Factors of Hyperuricosuric Male Stone Formers with High and Low Filtered Urate [23]

Using a similar approach to study 2 for hypercalciuric men, we investigated 153 male idiopathic stone formers who had hyperuricosuria. [23] As for hypercalciuria, there was a wide inter-individual variation in the net reabsorption of urate (the difference between the amounts of urate filtered and excreted per 24h) at each level of filtered urate, and the net percentage of urate reabsorbed was lower than for normouricosuric men (Figure 4). These findings indicate that a reduced capacity for net urate reabsorption is a common underlying abnormality in hyperuricosuria.

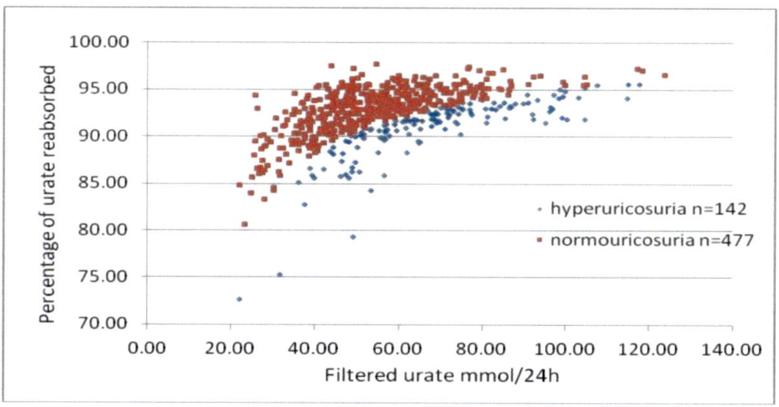

Figure 4. Correlation between filtered urate and net percentage reabsorption by 142 hyperuricosuric male stone formers with 477 normouricosuric stone formers after excluding those with clinical disorders or medications known to alter urate turnover. Spearman's coefficient r (95% CI): for hyperuricosuric men: r 0.89, CI 0.85, 0.92, P <0.001; for normouricosuric men r 0.70, CI 0.65, 0.75, P < 0.001. From Walker et al. 2014, Urolithiasis 42 (4) 291-300 [23]. Figure reproduced with kind permission of Springer Science + Business Media.

Thirty (21%) of the hyperuricosuric men had values for filtered urate which were below the median value for 477 male stone formers with normouricosuria. They were identified as a group whose hyperuricosuria was likely to be due to reduced net renal reabsorption of urate and were designated as low filtrators. In Table 7 their risk factors for stones are compared with those of the 30 men with the highest urate filtration ('high filtrators'). In both groups there was a high incidence of stone recurrence. Only 7% of high filtrators had a first degree relative with stones compared with 20% of low filtrators, but the difference was not statistically significant. In contrast to the findings in study 2 for hypercalciuria, there were no differences in age at the first stone episode or clinic assessment. However, there were differences in their factors for stone risk. High filtrators had higher urinary oxalate excretion, and low filtrators had lower $TmPO_4$ /GFR values. Calcium and urate excretion and urine pH were similar. Higher filtration was explained both by higher plasma urate concentrations and higher creatinine clearance. This was > 200l/ 24h in 75% of men. Most of the large excess of filtered urate was reabsorbed and 24h urate excretion of high filtrators was no higher than of low filtrators.

Mechanisms of Decreased Net Renal Reabsorption of Urate

Net renal urate reabsorption is decreased by medications, an expansion of plasma volume and genetic deficiencies of transport proteins for urate in the kidneys. We excluded patients taking uricosuric drugs, few patients had significantly impaired renal function (eGFR < 60 ml/min/m^2) and none had recorded inappropriate antidiuretic hormone secretion. [62, 63]

Renal Urate Excretion

Almost all the urate excreted in urine is produced endogenously as an end product of purine metabolism. It circulates in the blood as sodium urate which is filtered freely into the kidneys. In the proximal tubules, most of the filtered urate is reabsorbed into the blood but some is also secreted into the tubules. These processes occur in the proximal tubules. Normally around 8–12 % of the filtered load is finally excreted in the urine. [62, 64, 65] Urate reabsorption and secretion involves complex interaction between several transporters. Some have been identified and characterized. URAT1 is the major apical membrane transporter which reabsorbs urate. It is functionally coupled to two lactate transporters. The organic anion exchanger OAT4 also contributes to urate reabsorption. GLUT9 (isoform 1; coded by the *SLC2A9* gene) is thought to be the major urate transporter in the basolateral membrane which transfers urate into the blood and interstitial fluid. Another 10 or more proteins may also be involved in urate transport, in some cases coupled with transport of other anions including phosphate, oxalate, lactate and sulfate. [43, 66-68] Some, including URAT1 are tethered to a scaffolding protein, PDZK1, in the proximal tubules together with other transporters and these may function as a molecular complex. [43] So far, only two rare inherited deficiencies of renal urate transporters are known to cause heavy hyperuricosuria, in both cases with very low plasma urate levels: in URAT1 deficiency urate reabsorption from the renal filtrate is severely impaired; in GLUT 9 deficiency transport of urate from the proximal tubules into the renal interstitium is grossly reduced. [43, 64, 66, 69, 70] It is unlikely that any of our patients had these defects. As yet, no gene polymorphisms have been identified which are associated with hyperuricosuria. Variants of the *SLC2A9* gene associated with low fractional excretion of urate and gout have been reported. [65] There are numerous theoretical possibilities for interaction of transporters. For example, changes in ionization of anions (possibly triggered by abnormal H^+ secretion) might have a secondary effect on urate transport. Primary hyperuricosuria is likely to be polygenic in the majority of cases and due to the summation of inherited gene polymorphisms which individually have a weak effect.

Mechanisms Causing Hyperfiltration of Urate

Hyperfiltration in our study groups was explained by increased creatinine clearance and, in contrast to the hypercalciuric men in study 2, also to an increase in plasma urate. There was no evidence that the increased creatinine clearance was due to inaccurate urine collection in the hyperfiltration group as a whole. [23] A high protein intake could explain the increased GFR, and hemodynamic changes within the kidney might also reduce the renal reabsorption of urate (see the discussion above for hypercalciuric men). It could also explain the increased urinary oxalate excretion observed in the high filtrators. In one study, dietary protein restriction for 15 days reduced urate and oxalate excretion significantly, as well as decreasing calcium excretion. [51] The raised plasma urate levels of high urate filtrators compared with low filtrators may be indicative of a higher dietary intake of animal protein.

Conclusion

Kidney stones are pathological products. They indicate that there is a problem somewhere in the handling and/ or excretion of minerals or anions but rarely point to the cause. Hypercalciuria or hyperuricosuria are clues to the site of the primary problem but cannot identify it since they are merely biochemical end-points which may have multiple origins. In the majority of cases they appear to arise from a mis-match between the diet and the genetic constitution of an individual. Mineral absorption and excretion involves the interaction of numerous proteins, and polymorphisms of their genes will modify their activity. Family and population studies show that the inherited factors contribute around 50% to the risk for hypercalciuria, and that inheritance is polygenic. The capacity of an individual to handle minerals will depend upon the combined activities of the 'package' of genes inherited and their protein products. This in turn will determine dietary tolerance. With low capacity, hypercalciuria will develop even on a standard diet. The risk will increase with increasing dietary excesses. The escalation in stone formation world-wide is almost certainly a reflection of dietary changes. From our own studies we suggest that a higher protein intake may be an important contributor. With the dramatic recent developments in our understanding of mineral and organic anion turnover, and in technology enabling rapid through-put DNA analysis, we now have the opportunity to get to the root of the problems. However, it will be fundamental to define the phenotypes of stone formers as precisely as possible if the genetic analyses are to be fruitful. Stone formers could prove to be an exciting group for elucidating renal tubular transport mechanisms. Better understanding must surely expand the therapeutic options to prevent stone recurrence, which are currently very limited and have not progressed for decades.

Funding: The Southampton family study was funded by the then NHS Executive South and West. The data base studies were funded by the Southampton Hospital Charity.

Ethics: The Southampton family and data base studies were approved by the local ethics committee, now the Southampton & South West Hampshire Research Ethics Committee.

Competing interests: Neither author has competing interests to declare

References

[1] Coe FL, Evan A, Worcester E. Kidney stone disease. *J Clin Invest* 2005; 115: 2598-608.

[2] Hughes P. Kidney stones epidemiology. *Nephrology* 2007; 12: S26-S30.
[3] Robertson WG. *Urinary tract calculi.* In: Nordin BEC, Need AG, Morris HA, eds. Metabolic Bone and Stone Disease. Edinburgh: Churchill Livingstone, 1993: 249-311.
[4] Sayer JA. The genetics of nephrolithiasis. *Nephron Exp Nephrol* 2008; 110: e37-e43.
[5] Pearle MS, Calhoun EA, Curhan GC. *Urolithiasis.* In: Litwin MS, Saigal CS, eds. Urologic Diseases in America. Washington, DC: US Government Publishing Office, 2004; NIH No. 04-5512: pp 3-39.
[6] Tiselius H-G. Who forms stones and why? *European Urology Supplements* 2011;10: 408-14.
[7] Coe FL, Favus MJ. *Neprolithiasis.* In: Brenner BM, Rector FC, eds. The Kidney, 4th edn. Philadelphia: WB Saunders Company, 1991; vol 2: 1728-67.
[8] Tiselius H-G. *Aetiological factors in stone formation.* In: Davison AM, Cameron JS, Grünfeld J-P, et al. eds. Oxford Textbook of Clinical Nephrology 3rd Ed. Oxford: Oxford University Press, 2005: 1199-1223.
[9] Sakhaee K, Maalouf NM, Sinnott B. Kidney stones 2012: pathogenesis, diagnosis, and management. *J Clin Endocrinol Metab* 2012; 97: 1847-60.
[10] Levy FL, Adams-Huet B, Pak CYC. Ambulatory evaluation of nephrolithiasis: an update of a 1980 protocol. Am J Med 1995; 98: 50-9.
[11] Worcester EM, Gillen DL, Evan AP et al. Evidence that postprandial reduction of renal calcium reabsorption mediates hypercalciuria of patients with calcium nephrolithiasis. *Am J Physiol Renal Physiol* 2007; 292: F66-75.
[12] Frick KK, Bushinsky DA. Molecular mechanisms of primary hypercalciuria. *J Am Soc Nephrol* 2003; 14: 1082-95.
[13] Worcester EM, Coe FL. New insights into the pathogenesis of idiopathic hypercalciuria. *Semin Nephrol* 2008; 28: 120-32.
[14] Pearle MS, Roehrborn CG, Pak CY. Meta-analysis of randomized trials for medical prevention of calcium oxalate nephrolithiasis. *J Endourol* 1999; 13: 679-85.
[15] Moe OW, Bonny O. Genetic hypercalciuria. *J Am Soc Nephrol* 2005; 16: 729-45.
[16] Coe FL, Parks JH, Moore ES. Familial idiopathic hypercalciuria. *N Engl J Med* 1979; 300: 337-40.
[17] Pak CYC, McGuire J, Peterson R et al. Familial absorptive hypercalciuria in a large kindred. *J Urol* 1981; 126: 717-19.

[18] Curhan GC, Willett WC, Rimm EB, et al. Family history and risk of kidney stones. *J Am Soc Nephrol* 1997; 8: 1568-73.
[19] Griffin DG. A review of the heritability of idiopathic nephrolithiasis. *J Clin Pathol* 2004; 57: 793-6.
[20] Stechman MJ, Loh NY, Thakker RV. Genetics of hypercalciuric nephrolithiasis: renal stone disease. *Ann NY Acad Sci* 2007; 1116: 461-84.
[21] Walker V, Stansbridge EM, Griffin DG. Demography and Biochemistry of 2800 patients from a renal stones clinic. *Ann Clin Biochem* 2013; 50: 127-39.
[22] Walker V, Cook P, Griffin DG. Male hypercalciuric stone formers with low renal calcium reabsorption. *J Clin Pathol* 2014; 67: 355–60.
[23] Walker V, Cook P, Griffin DG. Characterisation of risk factors for stones in hyperuricosuric men attending a stone clinic. *Urolithiasis* 2014; 42: 291-300.
[24] Walton RJ, Bijvoet OLM. Nomogram for derivation of renal threshold phosphate concentration. *Lancet* 1975; 2: 309-10.
[25] Hess B, Hasler-Strub U, Ackermann D, et al. Metabolic evaluation of patients with recurrent idiopathic calcium nephrolithiasis. *Nephrol Dial Transplant* 1997; 12: 1362-8.
[26] Mossetti G, Vuotto P, Rendina D, et al. Association between vitamin D receptor gene polymorphisms and tubular citrate handling in calcium nephrolithiasis. *J Internal Med* 2003; 253: 194-200.
[27] Curhan GC, Willett WC, Speizer FE, et al. Twenty-four-hour urine chemistries and the risk of kidney stones among women and men. *Kidney International* 2001; 59: 2290-8.
[28] Rendina D, Mossetti G, De Filippo G, et al. Fibroblast growth factor 23 is increased in calcium nephrolithiasis with hypophosphatemia and renal phosphate leak. *J Clin Endocrinol and Metab* 2006; 91: 959-63.
[29] Prié D, Ravery V, Boccon-Gibod L, et al. Frequency of renal phosphate leak among patients with calcium nephrolithiasis. *Kidney Int* 2001; 60: 272-6.
[30] Prié D, Huart V, Bakouh N et al. Nephrolithiasis and osteoporosis associated with hypophosphatemia caused by mutations in the type 2a sodium-phosphate cotransporter. *N Engl J Med* 2002; 347: 983-91.
[31] Karim Z, Gérard B, Bakhou N, et al. NHERF1 mutations and responsiveness of renal parathyroid hormone. *N Engl J Med* 2008; 359: 1128-35.

[32] Prié D, Ureña Torres P, Friedlander G. Latest findings in phosphate homeostasis. *Kidney International* 2009; 75: 882-9.

[33] Telci D, Dogan AU, Ozbek E et al. KLOTHO gene polymorphism of G395A is associated with kidney stones. *Am J Nephrol* 2011; 33: 337-43.

[34] Schuette SA, Zemel MB, Linkswiler HM. Studies on the mechanism of protein-induced hypercalciuria in older men and women. *J Nutr* 1980; 110: 305-15.

[35] Suki WN, Rouse D. *Renal transport of calcium, magnesium and phosphorus.* In: Brenner BM, Rector FC, eds. The Kidney, 4th edn. Philadelphia: WB Saunders Company, 1991; vol 1: 380-423.

[36] Edwards NA, Hodgkinson A. Studies of renal function in patients with idiopathic hypercalciuria. *Clin Sci* 1965; 29: 327-38.

[37] Peacock M, Nordin BEC. Tubular reabsorption of calcium in normal and hypercalciuric subjects. *J Clin Pathol* 1968; 21: 353-8.

[38] Moe OW, Huang C-L. Hypercalciuria from acid load: renal mechanisms. *J Nephrol* 2006; 19 Suppl 9: S53-61.

[39] Borghi L, Schianchi T, Meschi T et al. Comparison of two diets for the prevention of recurrent stones in idiopathic hypercalciuria. *N Engl J Med* 2002; 346: 77-84.

[40] Lavan JN, Neale FC, Posen S. Urinary calculi: Clinical, biochemical and radiological studies in 619 patients. Med J Aust 1971; 2 : 1049-61

[41] Eggerman T. Review: genetics of urolithiasis European Medical Journal 2014. emjreviews.com/wp-content/uploads/Review-Genetics-of-Urolithiasis (accessed 29 12 2014).

[42] Weinman EJ, Mohanlal V, Stoycheff N et al. Longitudinal study of urinary excretion of phosphate, calcium, and uric acid in mutant NHERF-1 null mice. *Am J Physiol Renal Physiol;* 290; F838-43.

[43] Anzai N, Jutabha P, Amonpatumrat-Takahashi S, et al. Recent advances in renal urate transport: characterization of candidate transporters indicated by genome-wide association studies. *Clin Exp Nephrol* 2012; 16: 89–95.

[44] Sayer JA, Carr G, Simmons NL. Nephrocalcinosis: molecular insights into calcium precipitation within the kidney. *Clin Sci* 2004; 106: 549-61.

[45] Reed BY, Gitomer WL, Heller HJ et al. Identification and characterization of a gene with base substitutions associated with the absorptive hypercalciuria phenotype and low spinal bone density. *J Clin Endocrinol Metab 2002*; 87: 1476-85.

[46] Shenolikar S, Voltz JW, Minkoff CM et al. Targeted disruption of the mouse NHERF-1 gene promotes internalization of proximal tubule sodium-phosphate cotransporter type IIa and renal phosphate wasting. *PNAS* 2002; 99: 11470-5.

[47] Weinman EJ, Cunningham R, Wade JB et al. The role of NHERF-1 in the regulation of renal proximal tubule sodium-hydrogen exchanger 3 and sodium-dependent phosphate cotransporter 2a. *J Physiol* 2005; 567: 27-32.

[48] Ardura J A, Wang B, Watkins SC et al. Dynamic Na^{+}-H^{+} exchanger regulatory factor-1 association and dissociation regulate parathyroid hormone receptor trafficking at membrane microdomains. *J Biol Chem* 2011; 286: 35020-9.

[49] Levey AS, Madaio MP, Perrone RD. *Laboratory assessment of renal disease: clearance, urinalysis, and renal biopsy.* In: Brenner BM, Rector FC, eds. The Kidney, 4th edn. Philadelphia:W.B. Saunders Company, 1991; vol 1: 919-68.

[50] Hess B, Ackermann D, Essig M et al. Renal mass and serum calcitriol in male idiopathic calcium renal stone formers: role of protein intake. *J Endocrinol & Metab* 1995; 80: 1916-21.

[51] Giannini S, Nobile M, Sartori L, et al. Acute effects of moderate dietary protein restriction in patients with idiopathic hypercalciuria and calcium nephrolithiasis. *Am J Clin Nutr* 1999; 69: 267-71.

[52] Kim Y, Linkswiler HE. Effect of level of protein intake on calcium metabolism and on parathyroid and renal function in the adult human male. *J Nutr* 1979; 109: 1399–1404.

[53] Hegsted M, Linkswiler HM. Long-term effects of level of protein intake on calcium metabolism in young adult women. *J Nutr* 1981; 111: 244–51.

[54] Bosch JP, Saccaggi A, Lauer A et al. Renal functional reserve in humans. Effect of protein intake on glomerular function rate. *Am J Med* 1983; 75: 943-50.

[55] Krishna GG, Newell G, Miller E et al. Protein-induced glomerular hyperfiltration: role of hormonal factors. *Kidney Int* 1988; 33: 578–83.

[56] Tolins JP, Raij L. Effects of amino acid infusion on renal hemodynamics. Role of endothelium-derived relaxing factor. *Hypertension* 1991; 17: 1045-51.

[57] King AJ, Levey AS. Dietary protein and renal function. *J Am Soc Nephrol* 1993; 3: 1723-37.

[58] Walker V. Ammonia metabolism and hyperammonemic disorders. *Advances in Clinical Chemistry* 2014; 67: 73-150.
[59] Erez A, Nagamani SCS, Shchelochkov OA et al. Requirement of argininosuccinate lyase for systemic nitric oxide production. *Nat Med* 2011; 17: 1619–26.
[60] Kerstetter JE, O'Brien KO, Insogna KL. Dietary protein, calcium metabolism, and skeletal homeostasis revisited. *Am J Clin Nutr* 2003; 78 (suppl): 584S-92S.
[61] Margen S, Chu J-Y, Kaufmann NA et al. Studies in calcium metabolism. I.The calciuretic effect of dietary protein. *Am J Clin Nutr* 1974; 27: 584-9.
[62] Shekarriz B, Stoller M. Uric acid nephrolithiasis: current concepts and controversies. *J Urol* 2002; 168: 1307–14.
[63] Fenske W, Störk S, Koschker A-C et al. Value of fractional uric acid excretion in differential diagnosis of hyponatremic patients on diuretics. *J Clin Endocrinol Metab* 2008; 93: 2991–97.
[64] Tasic V, Hynes AM, Kitamura K et al. Clinical and functional characterization of URAT1 variants. *PLoS One* 2011; 6(12): e28641. doi:10.1371/journal.pone.0028641.
[65] Wright AF, Rudan I, Hastie ND, et al. A 'complexity' of urate transporters. *Kidney Int* 2010; 78: 446-52.
[66] Bobulescu IA, Moe OW. Renal transport of uric acid: evolving concepts and uncertainties. Adv Chronic Kidney Dis 2012; 19: 358–71.
[67] Eraly SA, Vallon V, Rieg T et al. Multiple organic anion transporters contribute to net renal excretion of uric acid. *Physiol Genomics* 2008; 33: 180–92.
[68] Wu W, Dnyanmote AV, Nigam SK. Remote communication through solute carriers and ATP binding cassette drug transporter pathways: an update on the remote sensing and signaling hypothesis. *Mol Pharmacol* 2011; 79: 795–805.
[69] Enomoto A, Kimura H, Chairoungdua A et al. Molecular identification of a renal urate anion exchanger that regulates blood urate levels. *Nature* 2002; 417:447–52.
[70] Vitart V, Rudan I, Hayward C et al. SLC2A9 is a newly identified urate transporter influencing serum urate concentration, urate excretion and gout. *Nat Genet* 2008; 40: 437–42.

In: Nephrolithiasis
Editor: Melody Shneider

ISBN: 978-1-63482-134-6

Chapter V

Contemporary Prevention Strategies for Nephrolithiasis: A Risk Stratification Approach

Andreas Bourdoumis, and Theodora Stasinou
Royal Devon and Exeter NHS Foundation Trust, Exeter, UK

Abstract

Lithiasis of the urinary tract is nowadays recognized as a significant health care issue, affecting millions of people worldwide and resulting in hospital admissions, medication prescription, elaborate surgical treatment and loss of working hours. Although major advances and innovations have taken place in the field of active stone management, there is little progress in the field of preventative measures. Recurrent stone formers, i.e., patients who most likely suffer from metabolic stone disease, are particularly affected, as practices vary amongst physicians and institutions.

In this chapter, we shall attempt to look into a risk factor-oriented approach to the contemporary preventative strategies in urolithiasis. Following a preliminary introduction into the epidemiology and pathogenesis of the disease, we shall present an individualized strategy for the various categories of metabolic and non metabolic stone formers, in a coherent and systematic fashion. We shall outline the importance of an integrated metabolic stone unit in tertiary care centers, by describing the structure and function of a state of the art unit and also emphasize on desirable outcomes.

Introduction

Lithiasis of the urinary tract is nowadays recognized as a significant health care issue, affecting millions of people worldwide and resulting in hospital admissions, medication prescription, elaborate surgical treatment and loss of working hours. Although major advances and innovations have taken place in the field of active stone management, there is little progress in the field of preventative measures. Recurrent stone formers, i.e., patients who most likely suffer from metabolic stone disease, are particularly affected, as practices vary amongst physicians and institutions. In this chapter, a risk factor-specific approach to prevention of recurrent urolithiasis will be presented. We shall outline the importance of metabolic screening and control in stone formers and try to provide some insight for what the future holds in general metaphylaxis of stone disease. The prevalence of stone disease has changed through time and knowledge of the latest figures is essential in understanding the importance of effective preventative strategies.

Epidemiology

Worldwide, urinary tract stone disease is becoming a growing issue, with a prevalence of between 2 and 20%. [1, 2] Prevalence of nephrolithiasis in the United States has doubled over the past three decades. This increase has also been noted in most European countries and Southeast Asia. [3] Racial and ethnic differences are seen in kidney stone disease, primarily occurring in Caucasian males and least prevalent in young African- American females. [4] In men, the incidence of kidney stones appears to rise after the age of 20 and peaks between 40 and 60 yr of age. [5] In women, the respective incidence rate is higher in the late 20s and decreases by age 50. [4, 5]

Nephrolithiasis has become increasingly recognized as a systemic disorder, [6] that is associated with chronic kidney disease, increased risk of coronary artery disease, hypertension, type 2 diabetes mellitus, and the metabolic syndrome. [7] It is a chronic illness with a recurrence rate greater than 50% over 10 yr, [8,9] and although largely asymptomatic at first, carries a

48.5% 56-year probability of symptomatic manifestations. [10] Lately, new data have shown a significant increase in the incidence of kidney stones in the pediatric population between 1996 and 2007, that was believed to be linked to the concomitant rise in respective obesity figures. [11]

Recurrent stone disease causes not only pain and distress in those affected, but also poses a significant economic burden from associated healthcare costs and lost working days. Minimally invasive lithotripsy, including extracorporeal shock-wave lithotripsy (ESWL), has revolutionized stone management, but significant progress in preventing recurrences is yet to be made. However, there is evidence that intervention in the form of lifestyle advice and some forms of medical therapy can reduce the rate of stone recurrence. [12, 13] It appears that metabolic investigation and prevention are important elements in the clinical management of renal stone disease.

Biochemical Principals and Risk Factors of Stone Formation

In any solution there is a relationship that expresses the degree of solubility of the solute. This is described by the solubility product constant (K_{sp}) for a given mixture at the point of saturation. At this point, some of the solute is continuously crystallizing out of solution, and at the same time, a similar amount of the solid dissolves into the solution. At the state of supersaturation, the solute concentration in solution is above that which would ordinarily result in precipitation if the solution were held at equilibrium. In the study of urolithiasis, the term formation product (K_f) is used to depict the saturation ion product point at which the spontaneous crystal nucleation will occur. If the concentration product is less than the solubility product, the solution is termed undersaturated, and crystal nucleation will not occur. The metastable region is the area between the solubility product and the formation product. Spontaneous nucleation may occur in this region, but further crystallization does not occur because of the presence of inhibitors of crystal formation. [14] A solution with a concentration product that is greater than the formation product is quite unstable, and crystal nucleation will occur spontaneously (Figure 1).

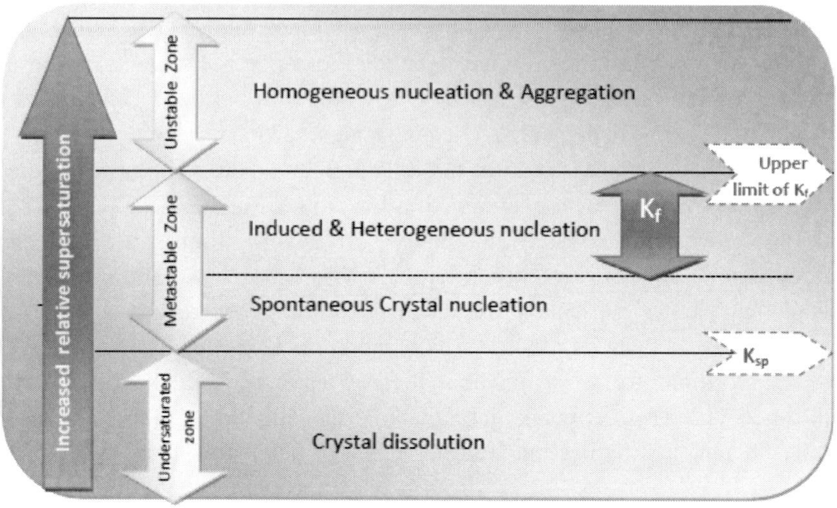

Figure 1. The biochemical cascade of stone formation. (K_{sp}: solubility product constant, K_f: formation product).

The above description constitutes the most widely accepted biochemical theory of initiation of stone formation. Nucleation is the first physical event in the cascade of urolithiasis. Two main theories have been developed to support the physical aggregation of the crystals into a solid structure, the free particle theory and the fixed particle theory. In the free particle theory, nucleation occurs as a result of spontaneous precipitation in solution. If supersaturation persists, crystal aggregation into clumps ensues. Both nucleation and aggregation can be either homogeneous or heterogeneous respectively. Hence the crystals grow or aggregate sufficiently within the transit time of urine through the kidney. Eventually, a particle will become trapped at some narrow point in the urinary tract and create a nidus for further aggregation and stone formation.

The fixed particle theory essentially refers to formation of Randall's plaques. Initial speculation revolved around subepithelial injury by ischemia or virulent factors and subsequent depositions of crystals in a supersaturated environment. Crystal adherence would be facilitated by the absence of crystallization inhibitors but also the presence of promoters (Table 1). This relation is the focus of intensive research and forms the basis of many of preventive strategies. The plaques originally described by Randall in 1937 are considered to form in the descending limb of the Loop of Henle as a result of urine supersaturation with calcium phosphate. [15] Subepithelial flecks of calcium phosphate are more frequently found in the renal papillae of stone formers than in those of individuals who do not have a history of urolithiasis. [16, 17] It is postulated that these plaques erupt through the papillary epithelium and expose it to various substances leading to the nucleation of a stone at the tip of renal papilla concerned. [18]

Table 1. Inhibitors and promoters of crystallization

Inhibitors of crystallization	***Promoters of crystallization***
Uromodulin (non polymerized form of Tamm-Horsfall protein)	Uromucoid (polymerized form of Tamm-Horsfall protein)
Citrate, Magnesium	Cystine
Nephrocalcin, Osteopontin	Uric acid
Urine pH (Alkaline > Acidic)	Urine pH (Acidic >Alkaline)
αAl and βnd microglobulin	Various urine glycoproteins

Table 2. Lifestyle/dietary and urinary risk factors for nephrolithiasis

Urinary Risk factors	***Lifestyle/Dietary risk factors***
Low urine volume	Obesity-Diabetes-Metabolic syndrome
Persistent Acidic or Alkaline urinary pH	Decreased water intake/Dehydration
Hypercalciuria	Low fiber diet
Hyperoxaluria	High protein diet
Hyperuricosuria	High Sodium diet
Hypocitraturia	High carbohydrate diet
Hypomagnesuria	High oxalate diet
	High/Low calcium intake
	Sedentary occupation/Stress

There are several risk factors that act as a substrate and form the ideal conditions for this complex biochemical interplay to come into effect and ultimately lead to a urinary tract stone. These can be classified into hereditary and acquired, anatomic and metabolic. The most important and recognised lifestyle/dietary and urinary metabolic risk factors and are summarized in Table 2. Obesity and high protein consumption are perhaps the risk factors that produce the most favorable conditions for urolithiasis, namely acidic urine, hypercalciuria, hyperoxaluria, hyperuricosuria and hypocitraturia. [19] The combination of the above with decreased water consumption and hot climate is probably one of the reasons for the increased prevalence of urinary stone disease in Arab countries and the Middle East. However, Western type diet, which is also high in protein and purines, has also been implicated in the development of metabolic syndrome and stone disease. [20-22]

It is important to note in addition that the broader spectrum of risk factors includes a positive family history of stone formation, especially for several inherited disorders of metabolism, such as cystinuria, primary hyperoxaluria, distal renal tubular acidosis, Dent's disease, Barttrer's disease and Lesh-Nyhan disease among others. Enteric hyperoxaluria (Crohn's disease/Ulcerative colitis, bowel surgery/ileostomy, sarcoidosis), medullary sponge kidney and hyperparathyroidism constitute special disease states that also predispose to particular type of stone. Urine outflow obstruction with urine stagnation and subsequent recurrent urinary tract infections that come as a result of an anatomical abnormality in the urinary tract (pelviureteric junction obstruction, calyceal divericulum, benign prostatic enlargement) deserve special attention and treatment.

Prevention of Recurrent Stone Formation

Initial Evaluation-General Measures

Contemporary prevention of nephrolithiasis begins with identification of risk factors during the first presentation of a patient with renal colic. An effective management plan should initially aim to completely remove all calculi from the urinary tract, either by medical expulsive treatment, shockwave lithotripsy or intervention. A complete stone free status is an absolute prerequisite for any future preventative strategy to have a reasonable chance of success. Even in severe, recurrent stone sufferers, such as in primary hyperoxaluria, primary hyperparathyroidism or homozygous cystinuria, reducing the stone burden and achieving a stone-free status is central to prevention in order slow down the rate of formation by minimizing the substrate available for supersaturation and nucleation.

Identification of metabolic risk factors and correct interpretation of results from 24 hour urine collection and stone analysis are central to planning an effective prevention strategy. The new Guidelines on Urolithiasis from the European Association of Urology (EAU) use a stratification system where patients are classified as low or high risk based on the absence or presence of risk factors mentioned earlier. Along with appropriate imaging, urine dipstick/microscopy and culture, full blood count, urea and electrolytes, ionised calcium and uric acid are the main initial investigations during the acute presentation. Low risk patients, i.e., first time stone formers without any risk factors, should be counseled to follow a general preventive measures plan for recurrences. The guidelines state that only high-risk stone formers require specific metabolic evaluation that should be guided by stone type. The recommended analytical procedures for stone analysis are infrared spectroscopy or X-ray diffraction. Thus, stone analysis is crucial and should be performed in all cases when a prevention strategy is likely to benefit the patient in the long term. [23]

It is important to stress patient compliance as a key factor to any preventive strategy. Adequate patient information regarding drinking and dietary recommendations plays a major role. A considerate approach in a dedicated outpatient setting and establishing good communication and a relationship of trust by setting realistic targets with the patient are essential elements to success. Lifestyle and diet modification is the primary approach independent of risk factors. Patients should be encouraged to mobilise regularly, lose weight to achieve a BMI of less than 25-27 (with respect to age, sex and body habitus) and manage conditions that lead to excessive fluid loss. A fluid intake of 2-3 liters of neutral pH, clear fluids per day, in order to produce a diuresis of at least 2 liters/day is pivotal to stone prevention for all stone formers. A limitation of salt intake to 4-5 gr/day, animal protein intake up to 1 gr/kg BW/day, normal calcium intake 1-1.2 gr/day (because of the inverse relationship between dietary calcium and stone formation) [24] and a balanced diet low in fats and carbohydrates and rich in fruit and vegetables constitute the general metaphylaxis plan. Lifelong commitment is necessary and should be explained clearly from the beginning. Appropriate lifestyle and dietary modifications should never be abandoned even when a pharmacological approach is started.

Low Risk Stone Formers

General metaphylaxis measures apply for all stone formers and constitute the main prevention for the low risk group. The EAU Urolithiasis guidelines recommend stone analysis in all patients at initial presentation; it is not clear whether this should guide further specific preventative measure sin low risk stone formers. However, from a more global perspective, a patient should be treated as a whole and not according to individualized findings. Therefore, it is reasonable to suggest dietary modification of i.e., animal protein and purine load in a patient with uric acid stones and suggest loss of weight and consider allopurinol if obesity and hyperuricemia are concurrent issues. Similarly, for the same patient, it would be questionable whether urine alkalinisation would help prevent further uric acid stones, or rather contribute in the crystallizations of new particles, like calcium phosphate.

High Risk Stone Formers

In addition to general preventative measures for all stone formers, patients with risk factors for recurrent and persistent nephrolithiasis deserve special attention. Initial evaluation should consist of the basic stone patient work up and also include thyroid and parathyroid function tests, urine spot test for cystine (Brand's test / cyanide –nitroprusside spot test) and 24-hour urine collection for analysis. For the latter, the patient should be provided with two (2) bottles (one plain - to analyse pH, electrolytes and urate - and one containing acid - to analyse calcium oxalate, phosphate, citrate and magnesium) of adequate volume to accommodate the urine and should be instructed to start collection in the morning of the chosen day after passing the first void. The collection should continue one bottle per day (including night voids) until the following morning, when the first void should be included. The patient should be instructed to use a clean glass or plastic container to gather the urine after voiding and then pour it into the bottle for collection containing acid. The results should be reviewed in a dedicated outpatient setting, preferably in the presence of a nephrologist with special interest in metabolic kidney disease and a specialized dietitian. The patient should stay on a self-determined diet under normal daily conditions and should ideally be stone free. A minimum of 20 days is recommended (3 months suggested) between stone expulsion or removal and 24-h urine collection. [25] High risk stone formers require specific dietary as well as pharmacologic intervention as part of their preventive management strategy. The stone type and the predominant metabolic abnormality should guide the choice of specific diet and medication.

i. Calcium Oxalate Stone Disease

Fluid intake of at least 2.5 liters/day is recommended to achieve a urine volume of at least 2.0 liters/24h. Mineral water with high bicarbonate (> 1,500 mg/l) and low calcium content (< 150 mg/l) should be preferred. Citrus juices are preferable beverages, but should be diluted with water. In predominantly oxalate stone formers avoidance of oxalate-rich food stuffs is recommended (chocolate, sesame seeds, spinach, rhubarb, beetroot, soya beans, tahini, tofu, nuts, peanut butter, okra, yams). Consultation with a dietitian might be required. Alkalinization of the urine with citrate containing agents plays a fundamental role in this setting. Citrate calcium chelation reduces ion-activity products of both calcium oxalate and calcium phosphate and inhibits growth and aggregation/agglomeration of these crystals, while increasing their solubility. Citrate supplementation is particularly important in patients with hypocitraturia and for bed ridden patients. Doses range from 5 to 12 gr daily for a period of no less than 3 months. Frequent urine pH and blood electrolytes measurements are required in order to avoid electrolyte disturbances and unpleasant side-effects, which range from mild gastrointestinal upset and diarrhea to hyperkalemia and cardiac arrhythmias. [26-32]

Hyperoxaluria merits special consideration. When isolated and identified in children or adolescent, it should prompt investigations for primary hyperoxaluria, a very rare hereditary disorder of oxalate metabolism, culminating to severe calcium oxalate nephrolithiasis and even death. In such cases, combined liver and renal transplantation provides a cure. Vitamin B_6 (pyridoxine) is used as a containment measure in these patients. Enteric hyperoxaluria is successfully treated with calcium supplementation 1-1.5 gr/day with meals, if previous intake l ess than 0.5 gr), citrate administration and magnesium supplements (200-400 mg/day). Care should be taken in cases of renal impairment, where magnesium is contraindicated. Management of hypercalciuria depends on the level of excreted calcium. For levels up to 8 mmol/day, urine alkalinization usually suffices. Idiopathic hypercalciuria is a common disorder in children and dietary modifications are often adequate. For levels > 8mmol/day, the addition of a thiazide diuretic is indicated. This effect is thought to be mediated by an increased reabsorption of calcium in the proximal and distal part of the nephron. [33, 34] Hydroclorothiazide is usually started at 25 and up to 50 mg dosage once daily. A supplementation with potassium citrate is needed to counterbalance the thiazide-induced potassium loss and hypocitraturic effect. However, treatment with thiazides has considerable metabolic side effects, such as development of diabetes and gout, and also erectile dysfunction, which contribute to a limited patient compliance (50–70%) and high dropout rate. [35-37]

ii. Uric Acid Stone Disease

Fluid intake of at least 2.5 l/d is recommended to achieve a urine volume of at least 2.0 l/24h. Mineral water with high bicarbonate content (> 1,500 mg/l) should be preferred. Citrus juices are preferable beverages, but should be diluted with water. Sodium reduction is advised, as well as reduction in animal protein intake and carbohydrates and loss of weight. Along with alkalinization, the addition of allopurinol is indicated in cases of hyperuricemia or hyperuricosuria (excretion >1.2 gr/day). Allopurinol is a xantine-oxidase inhibitor that prevents uric acid production from purine. It is administered orally at doses 100-300 mg/day. Care must be taken when administering allopurinol for prlonged periods. Reported side effects include Steven-Johnson or Lyell syndrome, vasculitis, hepatitis, renal failure and formation of xanthine stones. A new potential pharmacologic therapy for recurrent stone disease due to uricosuria is described by Goldfarb *et al.* Febuxostat, a nonpurine inhibitor of xanthine oxidase (also known as xanthine dehydrogenase or xanthine oxidoreductase) has recently been shown to lower urinary uric acid significantly more compared to allopurinol or placebo. [38] Febuxostat, at a daily dose of 80 to 120 mg, has also been shown to be more effective than allopurinol 300 mg in lowering serum urate. [39] However, a recent Cochrane review concludes that after 3 years of follow-up there were no statistically significant differences regarding clinical effectiveness and side effects between febuxostat 80 mg or 120 mg and allopurinol. More research is anticipated in this field and its particular role in preventing recurrent stone formation in hyperuricosuric patients. [40]

iii. Calcium Phosphate Stone Disease

Calcium phosphate stones are associated usually with alkaline urine pH. Apart from voluntary urine alkalinization for urinary stone recurrence, distal renal tubular acidosis (RTA type 1) can cause alkaline urine due to tubular defect in reabsorbing bicarbonate. Other causes include urinary tract infection and hyperparathyroidism. Fluid intake of at least 2.5 l/day is recommended to achieve a urine volume of at least 2.0 l/day. Mineral water with low bicarbonate (< 500 mg/l) and low calcium content (< 150 mg/l) should be preferred. Distal RTA can be corrected with pharmacologic interventions. Thiazide diuretics are used to lower urinary calcium levels, while L-methionine at doses of 600-1500 mg/day is used to achieve urine acidification. Aim is to reduce urine pH between 5.8-6.2. Hyperparathyroidism is usually treated with surgical removal of teh parathyroid glands.

iv. Cystine Stone Disease

Cystinuria is part of an inherited metabolic disorder of dibasic amino acid reabsorption in the kidney. While Lysine, Ornithine and Arginine are soluble is water solution, cystine is not, and excretion levels of more than 80 mg/day are capable of urine supersaturation. Heterozygotes excrete 200-400 mg/day, whereas homozygotes excrete >600 mg/day. It is known that 250 mg cystine will dissolve in 1 liter of fluid. For this reason, a large fluid intake of at least 3.5 - 4.0 l/d in adults is recommended to achieve a urine volume of at least 3.5 l/24h. Mineral water with high bicarbonate content (> 1,500 mg/l) should be preferred, as alkaline urine increases cystine solubility in solution. Citrus juices are preferable beverages, but should be diluted with water, due to the high content of oxalate. Urine alkalinization is indicated as a standard in cystinuria. Dietary advice concentrates around avoiding foods that contain high levels of methionine, such as red meat, fish and poultry. Further treatment involves the use of chelating agents that bind cystine to form soluble compounds. These include D-penicillamine, alpha-mercaptopropionylglycine (Thiola) and captopril. However, their use should be reserved for teh highly specialized setting of a referral centre that manages patients with cystinuria regularly, as there can be severe side-effects from inappropriate administration.

v. Struvite (Magnesium-Ammonium-Phosphate) Stone Disease

The prototype infectious stone is directly linked with urinary tract colonization with urease-producing Gram negative uropathogens that alkalinize urine and promote magnesium ammonium phosphate crystal precipitation. Fluid intake of at least 2.5 l/d is recommended to achieve a urine volume of at least 2.0 l/24h. Mineral water with low bicarbonate (< 500 mg/l) and low calcium content (< 150 mg/l) should be preferred. Primary control is to eradicate the infection and completely remove the stone burden. Prophylactic antibiotics are recommended according to sensitivity for a period of 3-6 months in cases of recurrent infections. This should be accompanied by regular follow up with imaging. Staghorn calculi rarely recur after complete removal, provided that a preventative strategy is followed postoperatively.

Conclusion

It is evident that recurrent urinary tract lithiasis represents but a manifestation of complex and sometimes genetic metabolic disturbances that require the involvement of a multidisciplinary team of experts in stone disease. This is ideally in the setting of a referral centre with a dedicate outpatient service that identifies high risk stone formers and initiates the necessary investigations for definitive management. Prevention is central in reducing the cost of urinary tract stone disease treatments. A recent study highlights the increase in prevalence and treatment of stone disease in the UK over the last 10 years. [41] This results in subsequent increase in healthcare spending as well as increased pressures on endourologic training and service delivery. A holistic approach is supported in order to achieve stone free status with minimal interventions possible while stratifying the risk and formulating individualized prevention.

References

[1] Buchholz NP, Abbas F, Afzal M, et al. The prevalence of silent kidney stones – an ultrasonographic screening study. *J Pak Med Assoc* 2003;53:24–25.

[2] Indridason OS, Birgisson S, Edvardsson VO, et al. Epidemiology of kidney stones in Iceland: a population-based study. *Scand J Urol Nephrol* 2006;40:215–220.

[3] Romero V, Akpinar H, Assimos DG. Kidney stones: a global picture of prevalence, incidence, and associated risk factors. *Rev Urol* 2010; 12: e86–e96.

[4] Lieske JC, Pena de la Vega LS, Slezak JM, et al. Renal stone epidemiology in Rochester, Minnesota: an update. *Kidney Int* 2006;69: 760–764

[5] Hiatt RA, Dales LG, Friedman GD, et al. Frequency of urolithiasis in a prepaid medical care program. *Am J Epidemiol,* 1982; 115:255–265.

[6] Sakhaee K Nephrolithiasis as a systemic disorder. *Curr Opin Nephrol Hypertens* 2008;17: 304–309

[7] Sakhaee K. Recent advances in the pathophysiology of nephrolithiasis. *Kidney Int* 2009;75: 585–595.

[8] Uribarri J, Oh MS, Carroll HJ. The first kidney stone. *Ann Intern Med* 1989; 111:1006–1009.

[9] Ljunghall S, Danielson BG: A prospective study of renal stone recurrences. *Br J Urol* 1984;56:122–124.

[10] Glowacki LS, Beecroft ML, Cook RJ, et al. The natural history of asymptomatic urolithiasis. *J Urol.* 1992 ;147(2):319-21.

[11] Sas DJ. Increasing incidence of kidney stones in children evaluated in the emergency department. *J Pediatr.* 2010;157(1):132–137.

[12] Hosking DH, Erickson SB, Van den Berg CJ, et al.: The stone clinic effect in patients with idiopathic calcium urolithiasis. *J Urol* 1983;130:1115–1118.
[13] Pearle MS, Roehrborn CG, Pak CY: Meta-analysis of randomized trials for medical prevention of calcium oxalate nephrolithiasis. *J Endourol* 1999;13:679–685.
[14] Johri N, Cooper B, Robertson W, et al. An update and practical guide to renal stone management. *Nephron Clin Pract.* 2010;116(3):c159-71.
[15] Randall A. The origin and growth of renal calculi. Ann Surg 1937; 105:1009–1027.
[16] Matlaga BR, Williams JC, Kim SC, et al. Endoscopic evidence of calculus attachment to Randall's plaque. *J Urol* 2006; 175:1720–1724.
[17] Matlaga BR, Coe FL, Evan AP, et al. The role of Randall's plaques in the pathogenesis of calcium stones. *J Urol* 2007; 177:31–38.
[18] Robertson WG, Peacock M, Nordin BEC. Calcium oxalate crystalluria and urine saturation in recurrent renal stone formers. *Clin Sci* 1971; 40:365–374.
[19] Chen HS. Increased risk of urinary tract calculi among patients with diabetes mellitus-a population-based cohort study. *Urology.* 2011;42(8):432–435.
[20] Del Valle EE. Metabolic diagnosis in stone formers in relation to body mass index. *Urol Res.* 2011;38(7):123–127.
[21] Maalouf NM. Metabolic syndrome and the genesis of uric acid stones. *J Ren Nutr.* 2011;21(1):128–131.
[22] Jeong IG. Association between metabolic syndrome and the presence of kidney stones in a screened population. *Am J Kidney Dis.* 2011;58 (3):383–388.
[23] Turk C, Knoll T, Petrik A, et al. *European Association of Urology (EAU) Guidelines Office.* Guidelines on Urolithiasis, 2014.
[24] Curhan GC, Willett WC, Speizer FE, et al. Comparison of dietary calcium with supplemental calcium and other nutrients as factors affecting the risk for kidney stones in women. *Ann Intern Med* 1997 Apr;126(7):497-504.
[25] Norman RW, Bath SS, Robertson WG, et al. When should patients with symptomatic urinary stone disease be evaluated metabolically? *J Urol* 1984 Dec;132(6):1137-9.
[26] Kurtz MP. Dietary therapy for patients with hypocitraturic nephrolithiasis. *Nat Rev Urol.* 2011;8(3):146–152.

[27] Rodgers A. Evening primrose oil supplementation increases citraturia and decreases other urinary risk factors for calcium oxalate urolithiasis. *J Urol.* 2009;182(6):2957–2963.

[28] Zerwekh JE, Odvina CV, Wuermser LA, et al. Reduction of renal stone risk by potassium-magnesium citrate during 5 weeks of bed rest. *J Urol.* 2007;177(6):2179–2184.

[29] Odvina CV. Comparative value of orange juice versus lemonade in reducing stone forming risk. *Clin J Am Soc Nephrol.* 2006;1(6):1269–1274.

[30] Kang DE, Sur RL, Haleblian GE, et al. Long-term lemonade based dietary manipulation in patients with hypocitraturic nephrolithiasis. *J Urol.* 2007;177(4):1358–1362.

[31] Zuckerman JM. Hypocitraturia: pathophysiology and medical management. *Rev Urol.* 2009;11(3):134–144.

[32] Caudarella R. Urinary citrate and renal stone disease: the preventive role of alkali citrate treatment. *Arch Ital Urol Androl.* 2009;81(3):182–187.

[33] Yendt ER. Renal calculi. *CMAJ.* 1970;102(5):479–489.

[34] Yendt ER. Commentary: renal calculi twenty years later. *J Lithotripsy Stone Dis.* 1990;2:164–172.

[35] Srivastava T. Diagnosis and management of hypercalciuria in children. *Curr Opin Pediatr.* 2009;21(2):214–219.

[36] Reilly RF. The evidence-based use of thiazide diuretics in hypertension and nephrolithiasis. *Clin J Am Soc Nephrol.* 2010;5(10):1893–1903.

[37] Huen SC, Goldfarb DS. Adverse metabolic side effects of thiazides: implications for patients with calcium nephrolithiasis. *J Urol.* 2007;177(4):1238–1243.

[38] Goldfarb DS, MacDonald PA, Gunawardhana L, et al. Randomized controlled trial of febuxostat versus allopurinol or placebo in individuals with higher urinary uric acid excretion and calcium stones. *Clin J Am Soc Nephrol.* 2013 Nov;8(11):1960-7.

[39] Becker MA, Schumacher HR Jr, Wortmann RL, et al. Febuxostat compared with allopurinol in patients with hyperuricemia and gout. *N Engl J Med.* 2005 Dec 8;353(23):2450-61.

[40] Tayar JH, Lopez-Olivo MA, Suarez-Almazor ME. Febuxostat for treating chronic gout. *Cochrane Database Syst Rev.* 2012 Nov 14;11:CD008653.

[41] Turney BW, Reynard JM, Noble JG, et al. Trends in urological stone disease. *BJU Int.* 2012 Apr;109(7):1082-7.

In: Nephrolithiasis
Editor: Melody Shneider
ISBN: 978-1-63482-134-6

Chapter VI

Nephrolithiasis in Polycystic Kidney Disease: Risk Factors, Treatment and Prevention

Alma Idrizi*[*]*, Myftar Barbullushi, Marsida Kasa, Nereida Spahia, Enton Kaçulini, Merita Rroji, Saimir Seferi, Erjola Bolleku, Xhoana Xhaferri and Alketa Koroshi

[1]Department of Internal Medicine, Service of Nephrology,
University Hospital Center "Mother Teresa",
Tirana, Albania

Abstract

Nephrolithiasis is an important manifestation of autosomal dominant polycystic kidney disease (ADPKD), which ranges from 8% to 36% in different studies. It is a frequent cause of morbidity because of flank pain, hematuria, and urinary tract infections. Nephrolithiasis is as common in females as in males and is asymptomatic in 50% of patients. Half of polycystic kidney disease patients are symptomatic and 20% require

[*] Corresponding author: Alma Idrizi, 372 Dibra Street, Tirana, Albania, Tel: +355684063625/ Fax: +35542363644, E-mail: almaidrizi@gmail.com.

surgical removal of the stones. Thc ctiology of stone disease in ADPKD is multifactorial, including both anatomic abnormalities (large, obstructing cysts and dilated tubular lumens may create tubular stasis, which predisposes to stone formation) and metabolic factors (hypocytraturia, hyperuricosuria, hyperuricemia and low urine pH). Also, in this high frequency contribute some risk factors such socioeconomic status of patients, geographic zones and dietary habits (most of them were from rural areas, consuming less water, more vegetable and animal proteins). Patients with a larger kidney volume predominant cyst size are at a higher risk of stone formation. Because of patients with ADPKD have a frequent occurrence of renal calcifications, the CT scan provides an excellent technique for detecting calcifications and for distinguishing renal calculi from cyst calcifications in patients with ADPKD. In ADPKD patients, the principles of management of kidney stones are the same as in patients with normal kidneys: percutaneous nephrolithotomy, while shock wave lithotripsy and open surgery are only indicated on few conditions. After removal of kidney stones, risk factors evaluation and control should always be considered to prevent or to reduce the frequency of recurrent stone disease in such patients.

Introduction

Approximately 4-6 million people world-wide suffer from Autosomal Dominant Polycystic Kidney Disease (ADPKD). It's the most common hereditary kidney disease and an important cause of end stage renal disease account for 7-10 % of people who are in dialysis or had kidney transplantation [1].

After decades with stable renal function because of a compensatory hyperfiltration of the surviving nephrons, patients may start the declining of renal function when greater than 50% of functioning parenchyma has been destroyed [2]. Nephrolithiasis is an important manifestation of ADPKD (Table 1), which ranges from 8% to 36% in different studies [3-11], about twice higher than in general population.

Idrizi et al. find this association to be higher than in other studies, nearly 42%, related to the fact that Albania is in an area of endemic urinary stone disease [12]. Most ADPKD patients affected by nephrolithiasis are above 40 years old. The disease frequency begins to rise between 20-40 years, making very uncommon finding nephrolithiasis under the age of 20 years [13, 14]; even so there are studies that have found cases of nephrolithiasis in ADPKD under the age of 20 years [11, 15].

Table 1. Clinical manifestations of ADPKD

Manifestations	Prevalence (%)
Renal	
Hypertension	60 before renal failure
	90 at ESRD
Pain (acute and chronic)	60
Gross hematuria	50
Urinary tract infection	Men 20; women 70
Calculus	**20**
Renal failure	≊50 by age 70
Hepatobiliary	
Asymptomatic liver cysts	80 at age 60
Symptomatic polycystic liver disease	Uncommon (male : female ratio 1 : 10)
Congenital hepatic fibrosis	Rare
Caroli disease	Rare
Cardiovascular	
Mitral valve prolapse	25
Intracranial aneurysm	8
Intracranial dolichoectasia	2
Ascending aortic dissection	Rare
Other	
Pancreatic cyst	9
Arachnoid cyst	8
Hernia	Rare
Inguinal	13
Umbilical	7

ADPKD - Autosomal dominant polycystic kidney disease, ESRD - end stage renal disease.

Nephrolithiasis is as common in females as in males. Half of ADPKD patients with kidney stone are symptomatic and 20% of them will need urological intervention [6, 8, 12]. It is a frequent cause of morbidity because of flank pain, hematuria, and urinary tract infections, hastening renal failure in these patients [5, 15]. Studies have found that ADPKD patients with lithiasis suffer more from low back pain that those without lithiasis [7, 8, 11]. So always consider lithiasis in ADPKD patients with flank pain. Hematuria is a frequent complication of lithiasis and ADPKD, increasing the risk of progressing into renal failure in these patients. In our study 65% of ADPKD patients with lithiasis have hematuria [15].

Risk Factors

Recent reports suggest that the etiology of stone disease in ADPKD is multifactorial in nature, including both anatomic and metabolic factors, and a combination of these factors [8, 9, 11, 13, 14, 16].

Intrinsic Factors

Anatomic Abnormalities

There are several risk factors which increase the potential of a susceptible individual to develop stones and one of them is anatomical anomalies in the kidneys. The structural abnormalities include cyst growth, obstructing cysts and dilated tubular lumens that may create tubular stasis, which predisposes to stone formation.

Nishiura et al. found that in ADPKD patients with normal renal function, higher kidney volume means higher risk for stone formation [11]. He observed that a renal volume of 500 ml was the only significant predictor of nephrolithiasis in these patients. So, while Grantham et al. [2] have shown that renal volume was related with proteinuria, microalbuminuria, hypertension, hematuria and progressive loss of renal function, Nishiura et al. suggest that greater kidney volumes are also associated with nephrolithiasis. Torres [8] and Grampsas [17] have previously reported that a significant higher number of cysts and larger predominant cyst size are observed in stone-forming ADPKD patients, suggesting the intrarenal anatomic obstruction as a cause for nephrolithiasis.

Metabolic Factors

The metabolic abnormalities include hypocitraturia, hyperuricosuria, hyperuricemia and low urine pH. The low urinary pH can contribute on formation of stones from uric acid.

Metabolic factors are equally important in the stone forming process as are anatomical anomalies in ADPKD. Gambaro et al. observed that metabolic disturbances were more frequent in stone-forming patients with renal anatomical anomalies [9].

It is important to categorize the stone-forming ADPKD patients in to two groups: those with normal renal function and those with stage 3-5 of CKD, before analyzing metabolic disturbances, because the presence of low renal function compromises the results of the lithogenic parameters [18].

Uric acid and calcium stones are the most frequent types of stones in ADPKD patients even though hyperuricosuria and hypercalciuria do not occur consistently in ADPKD patients [8, 12]. Umbreit et al. in his study also found that 55% of treated stones in ADPKD were primarily uric acid calculi [19]. Meanwhile, Daudon found that uric acid stones are the predominant type in cystic renal abnormalities [20]. The reason for this predominance of uric stones in this kind of patients is still a debate because of the low prevalence of hyperuricosuria (18-28%) [6, 15] in ADPKD with normal renal function and more over the lack of statistically difference in uricosuria between ADPKD patients with or without lithiasis [11]. In ADPKD uric acid homeostasis is preserved as long as the patient has normal renal function [21]. Different studies have suggested that more over than a disturbance in uric acid homeostasis, the uric acid lithiasis with normouricosuria is a renal acidification disease [22]. The same defect in urinary acidification and ammonium excretion is reported in ADPKD patients by Preuss and Torres [23, 24]. This abnormality is described as an inability to excrete adequate amounts of ammonium during acid overload, making the urine acidic. Nishiura et al. reported lower ammonium excretion after acid load in ADPKD patients with lithiasis compared with those without lithiasis [2]. It is obvious that acidic urine in these patients favors precipitation of uric crystals, making the uric stone one of the most frequent type in ADPKD patients.

Torres [6] and Nishiura [2] reported that hyperoxaluria was significantly higher in ADPKD patients with nephrolithiasis versus ADPKD patients without nephrolithiasis. The reason for this high frequency of hyperoxaluria is not clear.

Gambaro [9] found low levels of urinary phosphate, magnesium and potassium in kidney stone forming ADPKD patients while Nishiura observed no difference between two groups [2].

Hypocitraturia is a still unexplained feature of ADPKD and there is no statistical difference between levels found in ADPKD with or without lithiasis [6, 11, 17]. According to Torres, hypocitraturia and low urine pH are the most common abnormalities in ADPKD patients [8, 24].

Hypercalciuria do not occur frequently in patients with ADPKD and lithiasis, however calcium stone are very common as are uric stone in ADPKD patients [11, 15].

Other features of urine produced by ADPKD patients with lithiasis are the lack of ability to maximally concentrate urine and the significantly low urinary volumes [17, 23].

Staghorn calculus is a type of stone with very low frequency in ADPKD but with a grim prognosis. Urinary tract infection (UTI) is well-known as a risk factor for staghorn calculus, making the infection stone the predominant type in this case [25], but recently Viprakasit et al. found calcium phosphate calculus as the most common stone in his ADPKD patients with staghorn calculosis prompting for carefully metabolic evaluation in these patients [26].

Non Intrinsic Factors

Also, in the high frequency of nephrolithiasis in ADPKD patients contribute some non intrinsic factors such socioeconomic status of patients, geographic zones and dietary habits (most of them were from rural areas, consuming less water, more vegetable and animal proteins) [15].

UTI as a frequent complication occurring in 30-50% of ADPKD patients raise also the risk for lithiasis. The higher presence of UTI in ADPKD patients with lithiasis than without lithiasis is noticed in different studies [7, 11, 15]. With equal clinical relevance is considered also the asymptomatic pyuria in ADPKD patients, because of its potential for developing overt UTI, contributing this way not only in increasing the risk for nephrolithiasis but also in declining renal function [27].

Unconventional risk factors for lithiasis (calcium phosphate) are nanobacteria, which are microagents 100-fold smaller than common bacteria. They are considered now as powerful mediators for lithiasis and tubular calcification, also studies have found that human kidney cyst fluid contain nanobacteria [28, 29]. For now, we can speculate that nanobacteria may be involved in ADPKD lithiasis too, but further studies are warranted to determine their role.

Clinical Manifestations

The acute abdominal pain is one of the most important clinical manifestations in ADPKD patients, especially in those with nephrolithiasis (Table 2).

Table 2. Specific causes of acute abdominal pain in patients with ADPKD

Cause	Frequency	Fever
Renal		
Cyst bleeding	+++	Mild (<38°C, max 2 days) or none
Stone	**++**	**With pyonephrosis**
Infection	+	High, prolonged with cyst involved
Liver		
Cyst infection	Rare	High, prolonged
Cyst bleeding	Very rare	Mild (<38°C, max 2 days) or none

ADPKD - Autosomal dominant polycystic kidney disease.

The severe renal colic, which presents as severe flank pain, occurs in about 20% of patients with ADPKD [6, 8]. It is often an abrupt onset that peaks within 30 minutes and remains constant and unbearable and is associated with nausea and vomiting. The pattern of pain radiation may provide a clue as to where in the urinary tract the stone is lodged [30, 31]. Pain radiating around the flank and into the groin is common for a stone trapped at the ureteropelvic junction. Signs of bladder irritation such as dysuria, frequency, and urgency are associated with stones lodged at the ureterovesicular junction (the narrowest portion of the ureter) [32-34]. Pain may radiate to the testicles or vulva. Struvite stones are often incidentally discovered on plain abdominal radiograph because they are generally too large to move into the ureter. The abdominal, rectal, and pelvic examinations are directed at ruling out other potential etiologies of abdominal pain. Physical examination is remarkable for costovertebral angle tenderness and muscle spasm [30, 32]. ADPKD stone formers have larger predominant cyst size compared to non-stone formers [17]. Therefore, anatomic deformity related to cyst number, size, and growth may contribute to the formation of kidney stones, possibly through a mechanism of increased urinary stasis [8]. Since these therapeutic and palliative procedures may not be as efficacious, ADPKD patients may have to endure prolonged and repeated episodes of renal colic while undergoing medical management addressed towards the etiology of the stone formation. A rapidly progressive distension produced by stone movement usually causes a much more severe pain than a slowly increasing distension [35].

Renal prostaglandins may be a major contributing factor in the symptom complex known as renal colic. Acute ureteral obstruction by a stone can increase renal pressure, leading to a release of inflammatory mediating renal prostaglandins [36]. These prostaglandins, especially prostaglandin E_2 (PGE_2), cause vasodilation of the afferent arterioles in the kidney and inhibition of antidiuretic hormone (ADH), with a resultant diuresis and a further increase in renal pressure. Thus, a vicious cycle may be established [37].

Gross hematuria may associates the passage of kidney stones in ADPKD patients [3-5, 15, 21, 38]. The likelihood of spontaneous passage is 97% for stones smaller than 2 mm, 74% for stones 3 mm in size, and 50% for stones 4 to 6 mm in size; if the stone is larger than 6 mm, the chance of spontaneous passage is only 1%, and urologic intervention will almost certainly be required [15]. Gross hematuria rarely lasts for more than 7 days and blood transfusion is sometimes required. Very rarely, bleeding may be severe and persistent, notably in dialysis patients, necessitating uninephrectomy [22, 23].

Urinary tract infections are common in patients with ADPKD, especially in those with nephrolithiasis, causing sometimes fever (Table 3). As in the general population, women are more frequently affected than men [15, 39]. Computed tomography (CT) scan and magnetic resonance imaging (MRI) are useful to detect complicated cysts and provide anatomic definition, but the findings are not specific for infection. Nuclear imaging (67Ga or 111In-labeled leukocyte scans) may be helpful, but false-negative and false-positive results are possible [40]. An 18-F-fluorodeoxyglucose (FDG) positron emission tomography (PET) scan has become a promising agent for detection of infected cysts, but its use to diagnose kidney infections may be difficult because FDG is filtered by the kidneys, is not reabsorbed by the tubules, and appears in the collecting system. Cyst aspiration should be considered when the clinical setting and imaging are suggestive and blood and urine cultures are negative [40].

Renal function of adult ADPKD patients with kidney stones is significantly worse than in patients without stones [12, 17]. In a study of Idrizi et al. [12] the patients with kidney stones were compared as regard the renal survival with patients without kidney stones and there was no significant difference in renal survival between those patients (P=0.5) (Figure 1).

Table 3. Main causes of fever in patients with ADPKD

Renal infection (including cyst infections)
Upper renal collecting-system infection due to obstructive stone or clot
Liver cyst infection (rare)
Angiocholitis complicating biliary-tract dilatation (rare)
Colonic diverticulitis (essentially after transplantation)

ADPKD - Autosomal dominant polycystic kidney disease.

On the other hand, patients with kidney stones and gross hematuria had a poorer renal survival than those with kidney stones but without gross hematuria (median survival 44 years vs. 55 years, P<0.001, RR=2.8) (Figure 2).

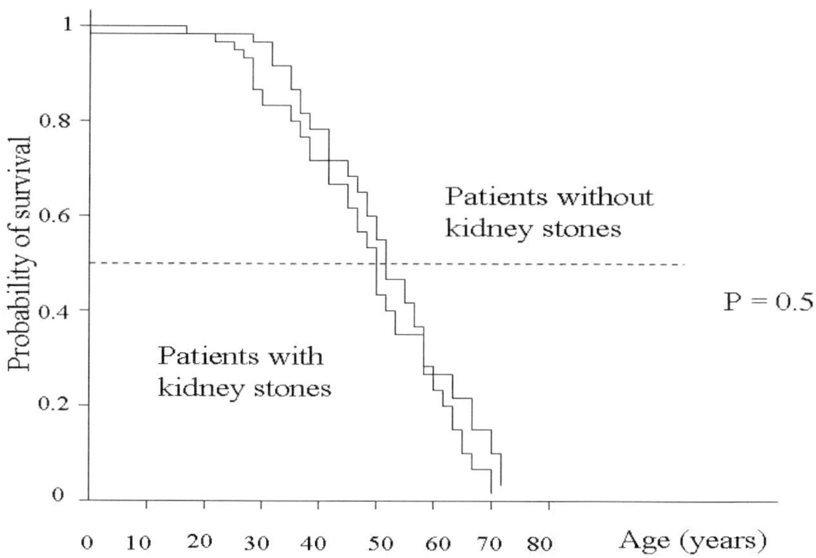

Figure 1. Comparison of renal survival between patients with and without kidney stones.

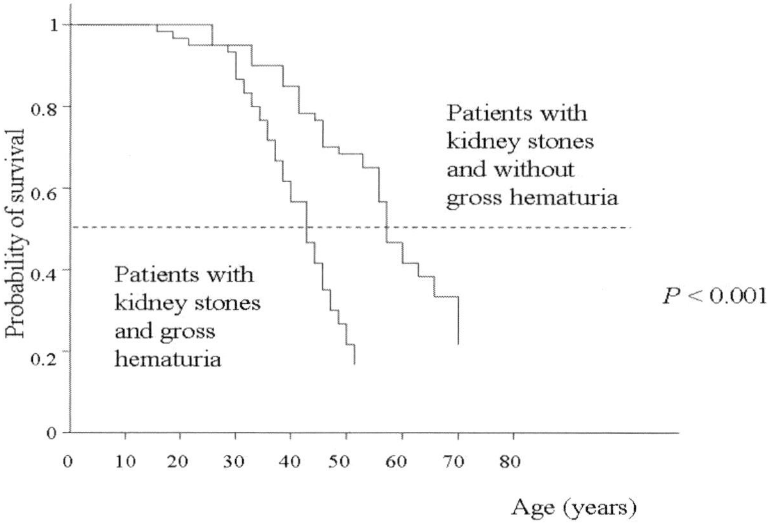

Figure 2. Comparison of renal survival between patients with kidney stones and with and without gross hematuria.

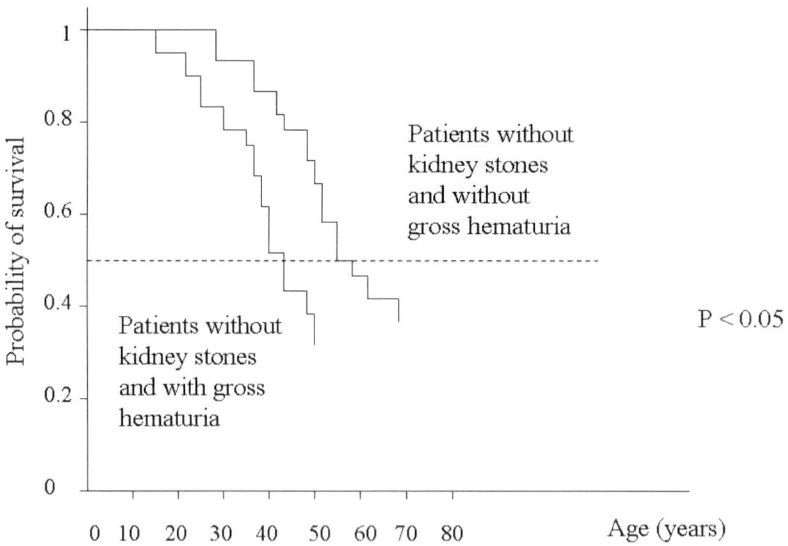

Figure 3. Comparison of renal survival between patients without kidney stones and with and without gross hematuria.

Also, there was a significant difference in renal survival between patients without kidney stones and with gross hematuria compared with those without kidney stones and without gross hematuria (median survival 43 years vs. 52 years, $P<0.05$, RR=2.6) (Figure 3).

Diagnostic Tools

Diagnosis of nephrolithiasis in ADPKD patients is difficult because of abnormal anatomy, cyst wall and associated parenchymal calcifications. Diagnosis of lithiasis in these patients needs the demonstration of the relationship of calculus to the complicated collecting system.

Imaging Methods

Renal Ultrasound (US)

Renal US is routinely used for diagnosing lithiasis especially for it low cost, but it's not always reliable (Figure 4). For stone smaller than 5 mm US have difficulties in detection renal lithiasis. When a stone visible on US is not detected with plain radiograph may be a uric acid or cystine stone. In ADPKD patients sometimes differentiate renal stone may be a challenge but when US is combined with KUB radiography can provide enough information to diagnose lithiasis. Nishiura shows in his study that when computed tomography (CT) scan is used as the reference standard, US has sensitivity 24% and specificity 90% [11].

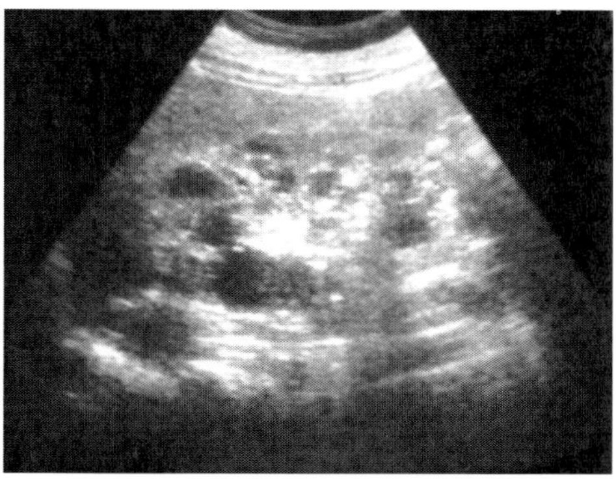

Figure 4. Renal ultrasound showing enlarged kidneys with multiple cysts and renal calculus.

Plain Abdominal Kidney-Ureter-Bladder Film (KUB)

It is a useful tool for assessing total stone burden and the size, location, shape and radiolucency of urinary lithiasis and also calcified cyst walls (Figures 5, 6). Because of stone composition, size or position not all calculus are visible on the plain radiograph, In ADPKD as a great portion of stones are uric acid calculi, plain X-ray KUB might not show all of them [8]. A large clinical study by Jackman et al. concluded that KUB is more sensitive than CT scan for detecting radiopaque nephrolithiasis. Of the stones visible on KUB, 51% were not seen on CT scan [41].

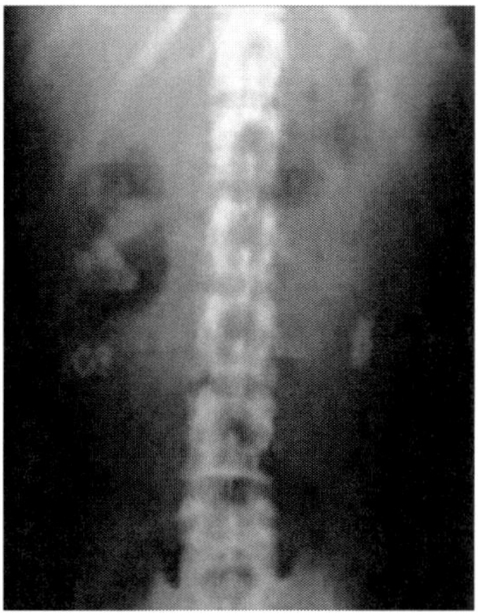

Figure 5. Bilateral renal stones on abdominal plain film.

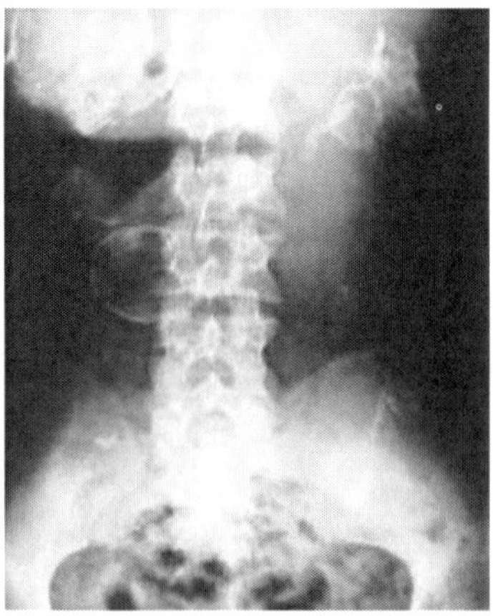

Figure 6. Calcified cyst walls seen on abdominal plain film.

The KUB radiograph can suggest the fluoroscopic appearance of stone, thus determining if the stone can be treated with Extracorporeal Shockwave Lithotripsy (SWL). When combined with CT scan, KUB radiograph can provide a better understanding of size, shape and location of stones and can help follow stone progress.

Intravenous Urography (IVU)

For many years is considered the standard criterion for renal lithiasis diagnosis. It is the most sensitive for visualization of entire urinary system [8] and in identifying the clear position of renal stone inside the collecting system (Figure 7). IVU is inexpensive but less sensitive than non-contrast CT scan. It was the test of choice for lithiasis before the introduction of helical CT scan. Nevertheless not all ADPKD patients can undergo IVU due to the associated kidney dysfunction.

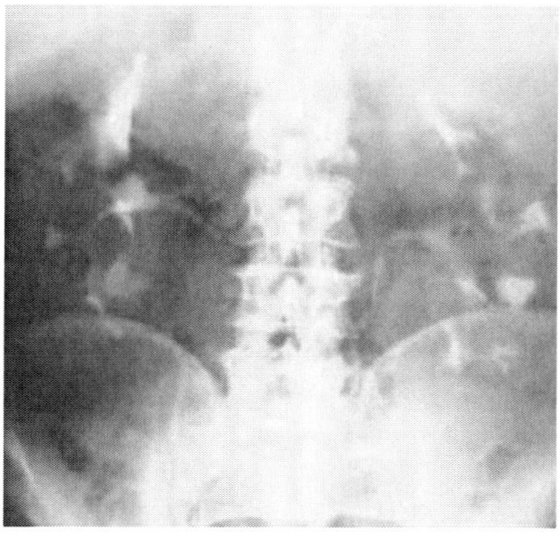

Figure 7. Intravenous urography in autosomal dominant polycystic kidney disease (ADPKD).

Plain Renal Tomography

It helps in difficult cases when more visual information is required for clarifying stones not clearly detected with other examinations, for example finding small kidney calculi [42].

CT Scan

It may be non-contrast helical (unenhanced) or contrast-enhanced CT scan (Figure 8). Unenhanced CT scan is a useful tool for detecting kidney stones, especially radiolucent calculus [7, 14]. Now CT scan is considered the most sensitive imaging technique for detection of lithiasis [8], being with superior sensitivity versus ultrasound. Nishiura et al. show the inability of ultrasound to detect the nephrolithiasis in 20 of 32 patients (62%) with CT scan positive for renal calculus. In his study he found a sensitivity and specificity for CT scan 63 and 81% respectively [11]. Cyst calcification occurs frequently in ADPKD especially in older patients. Distinguishing renal stones from these calcifications is often difficult using US, KUB radiography or unenhanced CT scan. Contrast-enhanced CT scan makes easier the classification of parenchymal calcifications into stones and cyst calcifications [7]. Stones may be missed if only a contrast-enhanced CT is obtained. Dual-energy CT can be used to distinguish between calcium and uric acid stones [25].

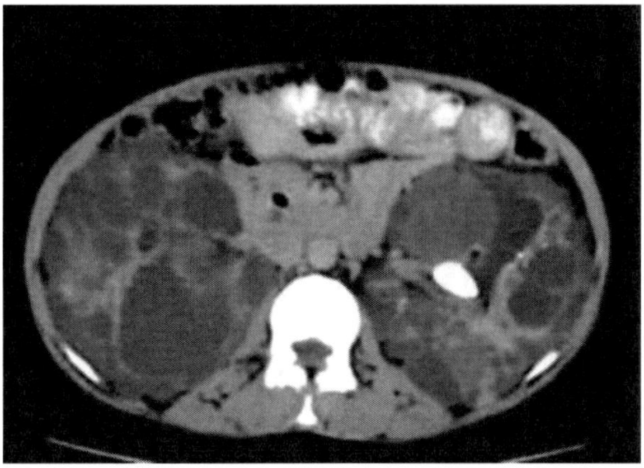

Figure 8. CT image showing enlarged kidneys with multiple cysts and renal calculus.

In the study of Idrizi et al. CT scan was better than ultrasound to detect urinary stones. 33% of patients with undetermined stones in ultrasound or KUB, presented evident images of them on CT scan [12]. Nishiura et al. have showed that CT scan for detecting urinary stones has a sensitivity and specificity respectively 63 and 81% [11]. In some cases a digital scout CT scan, formatted to look like a plain radiography can be used instead of KUB radiography for stone larger than 3 mm, but the scout CT scan sensitivity is not as good as plain radiograph.

In every case a detailed metabolic evaluation need to be done in ADPKD patients with lithiasis. For metabolic evaluation urinanalysis, urine culture, urinary pH, calcium, uric acid, citrate, oxalate, magnesium, phosphate, creatinine levels in a 24 hours urine specimen need to be performed in

ADPKD patients [9, 12, 15, 17]. In the study of Grampsas et al. the twenty-four-hour urinary analysis showed that patients with ADPKD and nephrolithiasis had significantly lower urinary volumes (P<0.05), and levels of urinary phosphate (P<0.05), magnesium (P<0.005), and potassium (P<0.05). Although not statistically significant, patients with ADPKD with stones tended to have lower levels of urinary citrate, and both groups showed a high percentage (range, 49% to 60%) of patients with hypocitraturia [17]. In the study of Idrizi et al. the stones were associated with an abnormal low urinary pH (5±0.3) in 72 patients (62%). In patients with nephrolithiasis hypercalciuria was found in 12%, hyperuricosuria in 42%, hypocitraturia in 43%, hyperoxaluria in 17% and hypomagnesuria in 23%. There was no difference in metabolic abnormalities between the patients with calcium oxalate stone and the patients with uric acid stones. In 60% of patients with kidneys stones (70 patients) the presence of stones was associated with a history of UTI and flank pain [12].

Treatment

Few decades ago open surgery was the only solution for treating these patients [12], now we opt for a team approach and careful tailored selection of the endourological procedures. Extracorporeal shock wave lithotripsy (ESWL) is the most commonly performed procedure [43, 44], however with the improvement of armamentarium flexible ureterorenoscopy (URS), retrograde intrarenal surgery (RIRS) and percutaneous nephrolithotomy (PNL) are considered now safe and efficacious options in the management of these patients. After removal of kidney stones, risk factors evaluation and control should always be considered to prevent or to reduce the frequency of recurrent stone disease in such patients. Treatment of lithiasis in ADPKD patients didn't differ much from lithiasis in general population. Small non symptomatic urolithiasis is treated conservatively, while symptomatic stone that do not respond to conservative treatment require interventional procedures.

Medication Management

Non-steroidal anti-inflammatory drugs (NSAIDs), prostaglandin synthesis inhibitors, would seem to be the obvious logical choice in treating pain from kidney stones. NSAIDs' administration leads to an immediate reduction in smooth muscle movement in the ureter as well as to a decrease in diuresis by counteracting the PGE_2 effects on inhibiting ADH [45]. Hetherington and Philip reported a 93% satisfactory pain relief from renal colic with intramuscular diclofenac in ADPKD patients [46]. Another study showed that a single dose of 10 mg of parenteral ketorolac was as efficacious as 100 mg of intramuscular meperidine in this setting [47].

We must avoid prolonged use of NSAIDs, especially in patients with compromised renal function secondary to ADPKD. Short-term use seems reasonable, limiting the NSAID administration to no more than two to three days [48].

Opioids are still the cornerstone of analgesic therapy for acute renal colic and in ADPKD patients, even though they do not influence renal prostaglandins or renal pelvic pressure. An increase in the tonicity of smooth muscle occurs with opioids and subsequent ureteral spasm during colic is not desirable [35].

Urological Interventions

The urological management of nephrolithiasis includes ESWL, PNL and surgical treatment [1–3]. Twenty per cent of symptomatic ADPKD patients with lithiasis will need urological intervention [6, 43]. There was time when open surgeries including nephrectomy were done for treatment of nephrolithiasis. In past few years these have largely been replaced by use of minimally invasive procedures such as ESWL and PNL.

Even having distorted intrarenal anatomy these patients can be safely and effectively treated with any or all contemporary, minimally invasive techniques, as we do in general population with lithiasis [8, 43]. Because of the compressed and distorted renal calices, treatment modalities such as ureteroscopy, ESWL and PNL are more difficult in patients with ADPKD [43, 44, 49, 50]. Because of this abnormal anatomy and the lack of sophisticated equipment, open surgery was the commonly used procedure in early reports in ADPKD patients with lithiasis [6]. Minimally invasive technologies as ESWL and PNL are used instead of open surgery for renal stone in general population. Rather than associated presence of ADPKD, size and location of renal stone determine the type of urological intervention [43]. Due to specific associated condition that accompanies ADPKD patients, before intervention attention is paid to correct electrolyte imbalance and to treat urinary infection.

A general rule exist for renal stone that those larger than 7 mm are unlikely to pass spontaneously and require intervention.

Surgical Options

Stent Placement

Internal ureteral stents when used for stone disease guarantee drainage of urine from kidney into bladder and bypass any obstruction, relieving patients from renal colic pain. Also stents dilate the ureter making the passage of ureteroscopy and other endoscopic surgical procedures easier. After large stones are broken up, stents tend to prevent the rapid accumulation of stone fragments and debris into ureter [43].

Percutaneous Nephrostomy

Percutaneous nephrostomy is useful in cases of obstructed kidney which need drainage, in particular when this obstruction is associated with infection [51].

Extracorporeal Shockwave Lithotripsy (ESWL)

ESWL is the least invasive method of surgical interventions, which utilize an underwater wave to break the stone into fragments. ESWL is a safe and effective method of treatment but less effective in large (> 2.5 cm) stone [5–7] and positioned in the upper or middle calyx [51]. Is contraindicated in pregnancy, untreatable bleeding disorders, very hard stones (cystine stones), in ureteral obstruction distal to the stone or in very obese people [52]. In ADPKD patients as in the general population ESWL is indicated for stones up to 2cm and can be used as a primary management tool with favorable outcomes [44, 53].

Ureteroscopy

Along with ESWL, ureteroscopic intervention is a frequently used method of stone removal which use a small endoscope most often a flexible one, who passed in retrograde from bladder into the kidney. It's mostly suitable for removal of stone 1-2 cm, positioned in lower calyx or those which are too hard for ESWL [51]. Ureteroscopic intervention is accompanied frequently with an internal laser therapy, called Holmium laser lithotripsy. The direct contact with the stone of Holmium laser makes it superior to ESWL [51].

Breda et al. found that in selected patients with single intrarenal calculus >2cm, flexible ureteroscopy (FUR) with holmium laser lithotripsy may represent a safe and efficient alternative treatment to standard PNL [54].

Studies have tried to determine the efficacy of FUR with holmium laser lithotripsy in the treatment of multiple intrarenal calculi and stratify this efficacy by stone burden <20mm and >20mm. The stone-free rates (SFR) for patients with a stone burden greater than and less than 20mm were 85% and 100 %, respectively [27, 55]. They found this procedure to be a favorable alternative to ESWL or PNL for selected patients with bilateral multiple intrarenal stones and also observed that it has lower SFR for lower-calyx stones, and higher SFR for noncalcium stones [56].

Percutaneous Nephrolithotomy (PNL)

PNL allow fragmentation and removal of large calculi through a percutaneous access. Due to its higher morbidity and side effects compared with ESWL and ureteroscopy, this procedure is reserved for large stones (>2cm) and in failed cases of ESWL [53]. In ADPKD patients, PNL as a method of stone treatment has been reported in few cases with limited experience [19, 57, 58].

Sometimes a combination of ESWL and percutaneous technique is required to completely remove all stones. This type of combination, called sandwich therapy, is reserved for large and complicated stone.

A large study of Osman et al. with 300 patients treated with PNL have demonstrated that performed in an experienced centre and under guidance of ultrasound, PNL is highly efficient procedure with no significant major complication for large stone [59]. Another study evaluated the role of PNL in management of ADPKD patients with lithiasis and noted that PNL is safe and effective method for treatment of lithiasis in these patients [57]. Umbreit report the largest single center cohort of patients with ADPKD treated with PNL for large or multiple upper tract calculi, and demonstrated its efficacy and safety despite the abnormal anatomy [19].

Baishya et al. [14] have advocated the ultrasound guided puncture and subsequent tract dilatation under fluoroscopic guidance. Bleeding remains a significant concern of PNL in ADPKD [19, 57]. The presence of multiple or large cysts, causing significant narrowing of the proper targeted calyx, could affect the approach and increase the risk of bleeding if forcible dilatation is tried. The compressive effect of cyst is more important than the size of cyst and their location to the target calyx. In such scenario, another favorable calyx then should be punctured to get entry in pelvicaliceal system and stones should be retrieved [14, 19, 57]. The PNL in ADPKD patients could be a staged procedure in which the puncture was done by a radiologist and later on the tract dilatation and stone retrieval by urologist [19, 57].

Intraoperatively the stone clearance can be enhanced by using the flexible nephroscope [57]. The residual stone fragments can be managed by ESWL for smaller stones [11, 44]. The overall success of PNL in normally located kidneys is in the range of 84-96.5%. Singh et al. found PNL success in 82.1% of patients [53] and the result of PNL with ESWL was 92.85% in other studies [59, 60]. The deterioration of renal function remains a concern of PNL in ADPKD patients. The renal trauma can cause loss of nephrons. Bleeding is a major concern in PNL with an average hemoglobin drop ranging from 2.1 to 3.3 mg/dl. As a result, 1-11% of patients overall and 2-53% of those underwent PNL for staghorn stones require blood transfusion. Most of the bleeding can be managed conservatively but it may require superselective angioembolization in 0.8% of patient [53]. The PNL in ADPKD patients is safe and effective procedure but the procedure is more associated with hematuria requiring sometimes blood transfusion, postoperative fever due to cyst infection and paralytic ileus [53].

In ADPKD patients, the principles of management of staghorn stones are the same as in patients with normal kidneys, however PNL can be challenging because of the distortion of kidney anatomy by cysts compression and the cysts can come in the way of puncture and need to be aspirated before procedure [10, 19, 25, 57, 61].

Team approach including the treating urologist and nephrologist is important. Preoperative correction of electrolyte imbalance is essential, and if required dialysis. Preoperative correction of urinary tract infection and urgent de-obstruction of the system may be performed if indicated. Careful selection of the procedure should be done in an individualized fashion. Additional puncture in PCNL can be avoided by a puncture wash. Vigilant follow-up of patients and patient counseling/education regarding the disease are important [14].

Retrograde Intra Renal Surgery (RIRS)

Baishya et al. performed this procedure in for residual stones following ESWL. The stones were broken with a Holmium Yag LASER at an energy setting of 10-12 watts. A double J stent was kept for one month. Both the procedures were uneventful with patients being stone-free one month after the procedure [14, 62].

Open Nephrostomy

Open nephrostomy now is rarely used (<1% of all interventions) since the progress made with minimal invasive procedures such as SWL and PNL. Disadvantages include longer hospitalization, significant blood loss [19, 57].

Nephrectomy

Baishya et al. performed nephrectomy in one patient with calculus pyonephrosis, when his fever persisted even after putting in a percutaneous nephrostomy tube [14, 63].

All treated patients after urological management need regular follow up with blood chemistries, urine examination, X-ray and ultrasonography of the KUB region.

Prevention

Risk factors evaluation and regular follow up should always be considered to reduce the frequency of recurrent lithiasis in ADPKD patients.

Conservative treatment of lithiasis in ADPKD patients consist in fluid intake, oral alkalization therapy and regular follow-up.

Fluid intake. Increased dietary fluid intake has been shown to have significant impact in primary [64, 65] and secondary prevention of lithiasis [66]. Also studies made in ADPKD patients have shown that decreasing urinary osmolality (U/osm) below that of plasma with the use of AVP-V2 receptor inhibitor (tolvaptan) was associated with reduced rate of cyst growth and slowing glomerular filtration rate (GFR) declining [67]. In ADPKD patients the same level of U/osm can be safely achieved by a daily intake of water of 3-4L [27]. So in ADPKD patients with lithiasis we have double reason to increase fluid intake to 3-4 L/day.

Oral alkalization. Most used alkalization agents are potassium citrate and sodium bicarbonate. Urinary pH should be maintained between 6.5 and 7.0. Urinary pH of more than 7.5 has the potential to precipitate calcium phosphate around the uric acid calculus, which would make it hard to dissolve.

Potassium citrate therapy plays a principal role in the conservative management of lithiasis in ADPKD, because of its beneficial effect in different metabolic abnormality that accompanied these patients.

It provides physiological and physiochemical correction of hypocitraturia and urine acidification defect also inhibits new stone formation in hypocitraturic calcium and uric acid lithiasis [68]. Studies have shown that potassium citrate may reduce stone fragments following ESWL [69].

Uric acid stone can be dissolved with alkalization therapy in most of ADPKD patients despite anatomical distortion [19]. Even very large uric acid stone can be dissolved in patients who have a high level of compliance with therapy. The usual dose to achieve the required pH is 15-30 mEq twice daily. However not all ADPKD patients will be suitable for potassium citrate therapy because of accompanying renal failure, high baseline serum potassium levels or because of associated gastrointestinal side effects.

Sodium bicarbonate can be used as alkalizing agent in cases when potassium citrate can't be applied. It has the advantage of limited cost but however must be used with caution in ADPKD patients with uncontrolled hypertension or congestive heart failure. The usual dose applied in lithiasis is 650-1000mg 3-4 times/day [70].

Conclusion

Nephrolithiasis is a frequent cause of morbidity in ADPKD population and given the importance of preservation of renal function in this subset of patients, a clear understanding of risk factors and management options available is with great importance for patient's outcomes.

The etiology of stone disease in ADPKD is multifactorial, including both anatomic abnormalities, metabolic factors or combined and also some risk factors such socioeconomic status of patients, geographic zones and dietary habits. Because of patients with ADPKD have a frequent occurrence of renal calcifications, the CT scan provides an excellent technique for detecting calcifications and for distinguishing renal calculi from cyst calcifications in patients with ADPKD.

In ADPKD patients, the principles of management of kidney stones are the same as in patients with normal kidneys: percutaneous nephrolithotomy, while shock wave lithotripsy and open surgery are only indicated on few conditions. After removal of kidney stones, risk factors evaluation and control should always be considered to prevent or to reduce the frequency of recurrent stone disease in such patients.

References

[1] Wilson P. D., Goilav B. Cystic disease of the kidney. *Annual review of pathology*, 2007; 2:341-368.

[2] Grantham J. J. Clinical practice. Autosomal dominant polycystic kidney disease. *The New England journal of medicine,* 2008; 359: 1477-1485.

[3] Segal A. J., Spataro R. F., Barbaric Z. L. Adult polycystic kidney disease: a review of 100 cases. *J Urol,* 1967; 118: 711-713.

[4] Milutinovic J., Fialkow P. J., Agodoa L. Y. et al. Autosomal dominant polycystic kidney disease: Symptoms and clinical findings. *Q J Med,* 1984; 212: 511-522.

[5] Delaney V. B., Adler S., Bruns F. J. et al. Autosomal dominant polycystic kidney disease: Presentation, complications and prognosis. *Am J Kidney Dis,* 1985; 5: 104-111.

[6] Torres W. E., Erickson S. B., Smith L. H., et al. The association of nephrolithiasis and autosomal dominant polycystic kidney disease. *Am J Kidney Dis,* 1988; 11: 318-325.

[7] Levine E., Grantham J. J. Calcified renal stones and cyst calcification in autosomal dominant polycystic kidney disease: Clinical and CT study in 84 patients. *Am J Roentgenol,* 1992; 159: 77-81.

[8] Torres W. E., Wilson D. M., Hattery R. R. et al. Renal stones disease in autosomal dominant polycystic kidney disease. *Am J Kidney Dis,* 1993; 22: 513-519.

[9] Gambaro G., Fabris A., Puliatta D. et al. Lithiasis in cystic kidney disease and malformations of the urinary tract. *Urol Res,* 2006; 34: 102-107.

[10] Mufti U. B., Nalagatla S. K. Nephrolithiasis in autosomal dominant polycystic kidney disease. *Journal of endourology / Endourological Society,* 2010; 24: 1557-1561.

[11] Nishiura J. L. et al. Evaluation of nephrolithiasis in autosomal dominant polycystic kidney disease patients. *CJASN,* 2009: 4: 838-844.

[12] Idrizi A., Barbullushi M., Gjata M. et al. Prevalence of nephrolithiasis in polycystic kidney disease. *Central European Journal of Medicine*, 2011; 6 (4): 497-501.

[13] Dimitrakov D., Simeonov S. Studies on nephrolithiasis in patients with autosomal dominant polycystic kidney disease. *Folia medica,* 1994; 36: 27-30.

[14] Baishya R. et al. Management of nephrolithiasis in autosomal dominant polycystic kidney disease - A single center experience. *Urology annals,* 2012; 4: 29-33.

[15] Idrizi A., Barbullushi M. et al. The influence of renal manifestations to the progression of autosomal dominant polycystic kidney disease. *Hippokratia,* 2009;13(3):161-164.

[16] Bajwa Z. H., Sial K. A., Malik A. B. et al. Pain patterns in patients with polycystic kidney disease. *Kidney Int,* 2004; 66: 1561-1569.

[17] Grampsas S. A., Chandhoke P. S., Fan J. et al. Anatomic and metabolic risk factors for nephrolithiasis in patients with autosomal dominant polycystic kidney disease. *Am J Kidney Dis,* 2000; 36(1): 53-57.

[18] Heilberg I. P., Boim M. A., Schor N. Biochemical differences between stone formers and normal subjects. *Stone Disease [1st International Consultation on Stone Disease],* 2003; 21: 61-64.

[19] Umbreit E. C. *et al.* Percutaneous nephrolithotomy for large or multiple upper tract calculi and autosomal dominant polycystic kidney disease. *The Journal of urology,* 2010; 183: 183-187.

[20] Daudon M., Cohen-Solal F., Lacour B. et al. Urinary stones and urinary tract abnormalities. Is the stone composition independent of the anatomical abnormality? *Progres en urologie : journal de l'Association francaise d'urologie et de la Societe francaise d'urologie,* 2003; 13: 1320-1329.

[21] Kaehny W. D. *et al.* Uric acid handling in autosomal dominant polycystic kidney disease with normal filtration rates. *Am J Med,* 1990; 89: 49-52.

[22] Sakhaee K., Adams-Huet B., Moe O. W. et al. Pathophysiologic basis for normouricosuric uric acid nephrolithiasis. *Kidney international,* 202; 62: 971-979.

[23] Preuss H. et al. Tubular function in adult polycystic kidney disease. *Nephron,* 1979; 24: 198-204.

[24] Torres V. E., Keith D. S., Offord K. P. et al. Renal ammonia in autosomal dominant polycystic kidney disease. *Kidney international,* 1994; 45: 1745-1753.

[25] Mao Z., Xu J., Ye C. et al. Complete staghorn calculus in polycystic kidney disease: infection is still the cause. *BMC nephrology,* 2013; 14: 168.

[26] Viprakasit D. P., Sawyer M. D., Herrell S. D. et al. Changing composition of staghorn calculi. *The Journal of urology,* 2011; 186: 2285-2290.

[27] Hwang J. H. et al. Chronic asymptomatic pyuria precedes overt urinary tract infection and deterioration of renal function in autosomal dominant polycystic kidney disease. *BMC nephrology,* 2013; 14: 1.

[28] Kajander E. O., Ciftcioglu N., Miller-Hjelle M. A. et al. Nanobacteria: controversial pathogens in nephrolithiasis and polycystic kidney disease. *Current opinion in nephrology and hypertension,* 2001; 10: 445-452.

[29] Shiekh F. A., Khullar M., Singh S. K. Lithogenesis: induction of renal calcifications by nanobacteria. *Urological research,* 2006; 34: 53-57.

[30] Elzinga L. W., Bennett W. M. Miscellaneous renal and systemic complications of autosomal dominant polycystic kidney disease including infection. In: Watson M.L., Torres V.E. Polycystic Kidney Disease, Vol. 1. Oxford, England: Oxford Medical Publications. 1996, 483-499.

[31] Ueno A., Kawamura T., Wgawa A., et al. Relation of spontaneous passage of ureteral calculi to size. *Urology,* 1977; 10: 544-546.

[32] Teichman J. M. H. Acute renal colic from ureteral calculus. *N Engl J Med,* 2004; 350:684-693.

[33] Segura J. W., Patterson D. E., LeRoy A. J. et al. Percutaneous removal of kidney stones: review of 1000 cases. *J Urol,* 1985; 134: 1077-1081.

[34] Segura J. W., Preminger G. M., Assimos D. G. et al. Ureteral Stones Clinical Guidelines Panel summary report on the management of ureteral calculi. *J Urol,* 1997; 158: 1915-1921.

[35] Bajwa Z. H., Gupta S., Carol A. et al. Pain management in polycystic kidney disease. *Kidney International,* 2001; 60: 1631-1644.

[36] Zwergel U., Zwergel T., Ziegler M. Effects of prostglandins and prostaglandin synthetase inhibitors on acutely obstructed kidneys in the dog. *Urol Int,* 1991; 47: 64-69.

[37] Van Laecke E., Oosterlinck W. Physiopathology of renal colic and therapeutic consequences. *Acta Urol Belgica,* 1994; 62: 15-18.

[38] Gabow P. A., Duley I., Johnson A. M. Clinical profiles of gross hematuria in autosomal dominant polycystic kidney disease. *Am J Kidney Dis,* 1992; 20: 140-143.

[39] Sallée M., Rafat C., Zahar J. R., et al. Cyst Infections in Patients with Autosomal Dominant Polycystic Kidney Disease. *Clin J Am Soc Nephrol,* 2009; 4: 1183-1189.

[40] Soussan M., Sberro R., Wartski M. et al. Diagnosis and localization of renal cyst infection by 18F-fluorodeoxyglucose PET/CT in polycystic kidney disease. *Ann Nucl Med,* 2008; 22(6): 529-531.

[41] Jackman S. V., Potter S. R., Regan F. Et al. Plain abdominal x-ray versus computerized tomography screening: sensitivity for stone localization after nonenhanced spiral computerized tomography. *J Urol,* 2000; 164(2): 308-310.

[42] Matlaga B. R., Kawamoto S., Fishman E. Dual source computed tomography: A novel technique to determine stone composition. *Urology,* 2008; 72(5): 1164-1168.

[43] Ng C. S., Yost A., Streem S. B. Nephrolithiasis associated with autosomal dominant polycystic kidney disease: contemporary urological management. *The Journal of urology,* 2000; 163: 726-729.

[44] Delakas D., Daskalopoulos G., Cranidis A. Extracorporeal shockwave lithotripsy for urinary calculi in autosomal dominant polycystic kidney disease. *Journal of endourology / Endourological Society,* 1997; 11: 167-170.

[45] Johnston H. H., Herzog J. P., Lauler D. P. Effect of prostaglandin E on renal hemodynamics, sodium and water excretion. *Am J Physiol,* 1967; 231: 939-944.

[46] Hetherington J. W., Philp M. H. Diclofenac sodium versus pethidine in acute renal colic. *Br Med J,* 1986; 292: 237-238.

[47] Oosterlinck W., Philip N. H., Charig C. et al. A double blind single dose comparison of intramuscular ketorolac, tromethamine and pethidine in the treatment of renal colic. *J Clin Pharmacol,* 1990; 30: 336-341.

[48] McIntire S. C., Rubenstein R. C., Gartner J. C. et al. Acute flank pain and reversible renal dysfunction associated with nonsteroidal anti-inflammatory drug use. *Pediatrics,* 1993; 92: 459-463.

[49] Anderson G. A., Degroot D., Lawson R. K. Polycystic renal disease. *Urol,* 1993; 42: 358-364.

[50] Chen W. C., Lee Y. H., Huang J. K. et al. Experience using extracorporeal shock-wave lithotripsy to treat urinary calculi in problem kidneys. *Urol Int,* 1993; 51: 32-38.

[51] Wolf J. S. Nephrolithiasis. *Medscape,* 2014.

[52] Pareek G., Hedican S. P., Lee F. T. et al. Shock wave lithotripsy success determined by skin-to-stone distance on computed tomography. *Urology,* 2005; 66: 941-944.

[53] Singh V., Sinha R. J., Gupta D. K. Percutaneous Nephrolithotomy in Autosomal Dominant Polycystic Kidney Disease: Is it Different from Percutaneous Nephrolithotomy in Normal Kidney? *Current urology,* 2013; 7: 7-13.

[54] Breda A., Ogunyemi O., Leppert J. T. et al. Flexible ureteroscopy and laser lithotripsy for single intrarenal stones 2 cm or greater-is this the new frontier? *The Journal of urology,* 2008; 179: 981-984.

[55] Breda A., Ogunyemi O., Leppert J. T. et al. Flexible ureteroscopy and laser lithotripsy for multiple unilateral intrarenal stones. *European urology,* 2009; 55: 1190-1196.

[56] Xu C., Song R. J., Jiang M. J. et al. Flexible Ureteroscopy with Holmium Laser Lithotripsy: A New Choice for Intrarenal Stone Patients. *Urologia internationalis*, 2014;7.

[57] Al-Kandari A. M., Shoma A. M., Eraky I. Et al. Percutaneous nephrolithotomy for management of upper urinary tract calculi in patients with autosomal dominant polycystic kidney disease. *Urology,* 2009; 74: 273-277.

[58] Srivastava A., Bansal R., Srivastava A., et al. Percutaneous nephrolithotomy in polycystic kidney disease: is it safe and effective? *Int Urol Nephrol,* 2012; 44: 725-730.

[59] Osman M. et al. Percutaneous nephrolithotomy with ultrasonography-guided renal access: experience from over 300 cases. *BJU international,* 2005; 96: 875-878.

[60] Shoma A. M., Eraky I., El-Kenawy M. R. et al. Percutaneous nephrolithotomy in prone and supine position: technical aspects and functional outcome compared with the prone technique. *Urology,* 2002; 60: 388-392.

[61] Ganpule A. P., Desai M. Management of the staghorn calculus: multiple-tract versus single-tract percutaneous nephrolithotomy. *Current opinion in urology,* 2008; 18: 220-223.

[62] Yili L., Li Yongzhi L., Ning L. et al. Flexible ureteroscopy and holmium laser lithotripsy for treatment of upper urinary tract calculi in patients with autosomal dominant polycystic kidney disease. *Urological Research,* 2011; 40(1): 87-91.

[63] Gupta N. P., Goel R., Hemal A.K. et al. Should retroperitoneoscopic nephrectomy be the standard of care for benign nonfunctioning kidneys? An outcome analysis based on experience with 449 cases in a 5-year period. *The Journal of Urology,* 2004; 172(4): 1411-1413.

[64] Curhan G. C., Willett W. C., Rimm E. B. et al. Family history and risk of kidney stones. *JASN,* 1997; 8: 1568-1573.

[65] Taylo E. N., Stampfer M. J. et al. Dietary factors and the risk of incident kidney stones in men: new insights after 14 years of follow-up. *JASN,* 2004; 15: 3225-3232.

[66] Borghi L. et al. Urinary volume, water and recurrences in idiopathic calcium nephrolithiasis: a 5-year randomized prospective study. *The Journal of urology,* 1996; 155: 839-843.

[67] Torres V. E. et al. Tolvaptan in patients with autosomal dominant polycystic kidney disease. *The New England journal of medicine,* 2012; 367: 2407-2418.

[68] Pak C. Y. Citrate and renal calculi: an update. *Mineral and electrolyte metabolism,* 1994; 20: 371-377.

[69] Soygur T., Akbay A. et al. Effect of potassium citrate therapy on stone recurrence and residual fragments after shockwave lithotripsy in lower caliceal calcium oxalate urolithiasis: a randomized controlled trial. *Journal of endourology / Endourological Society,* 2002; 16: 149-152.

[70] Ngo T. C., Assimos D. G. Uric Acid nephrolithiasis: recent progress and future directions. *Reviews in urology,* 2007; 9: 17-27.

In: Nephrolithiasis
Editor: Melody Shneider

ISBN: 978-1-63482-134-6

Chapter VII

Nephrolithiasis: Risk Factors, Treatment and Prevention in Autosomal Dominant Polycystic Kidney Disease

Neetika Garg[1] and Theodore I. Steinman[2*]
[1]Department of Nephrology, Beth Israel Deaconess Medical Center, Boston, Massachusetts, US
[2]Department of Medicine, Harvard Medical School, Boston, Massachusetts, US and Beth Israel Deaconess Medical Center, Boston, Massachusetts, US

Abstract

Up to one-third of the patients with Autosomal Dominant Polycystic Kidney Disease (ADPKD) develop nephrolithiasis; this prevalence is seven to ten-fold higher as compared to the general population. Additionally, morbidity related to stones is especially high in ADPKD – nearly half of the patients with nephrolithiasis have symptoms over the course of their lifetime and one-fifth of the symptomatic patients require urological intervention. Risk factors for stone formation in ADPKD are

* Phone number: 617-667-5278, email: tsteinma@bidmc.harvard.edu)

both structural and metabolic. In particular, more than half of the stones are of uric acid composition. With normal urate handling observed in this group, this propensity for uric acid crystallization is attributable to increased urinary acidification and lower urinary pH seen in ADPKD. One mechanism that may explain this finding is the stimulatory effect of an overactive renin-angiotensin-aldosterone-system, a consequence of local parenchymal ischemia from compression by expanding cysts on the α-intercalated cells in the collecting duct system. Although most surgical techniques, including extracorporeal shock wave lithotripsy and percutaneous nephrolithotomy, are effective in stone removal, the risks of complications and residual stones are higher in ADPKD as compared to those in the non-ADPKD population with nephrolithiasis. A high rate of stone recurrence underlines the importance of dietary and medical management for secondary stone prevention in this population. Clinical evaluation, including a 24-hour urine metabolic profile, is needed to determine the precise risk factors in an individual patient and for developing the appropriate strategy for minimizing future stones.

Our focus is on the various aspects of stone disease unique to ADPKD, including the reasons for high incidence of stones (in particular, uric acid stones); the nuances of diagnosis, evaluation and treatment unique to this population; and the different strategies for secondary prevention in affected patients.

Introduction

Autosomal Dominant Polycystic Kidney Disease (ADPKD) is the most common inherited cystic renal disease; it affects 1 in every 400 to 1000 individuals and is the underlying etiology in approximately 5% of the patients who initiate dialysis every year in the United States. Pain is common and occurs early in the course of ADPKD; it affects more than 60 percent of the patients and is frequently observed decades before the onset of renal insufficiency [1, 2]. The differential diagnosis of acute abdominal and/or flank pain related to ADPKD itself includes renal parenchymal infection (i.e., pyelonephritis), cyst infection (i.e., pyocystis), cyst rupture, hemorrhage into a cyst and nephrolithiasis. With regard to the latter, 20 to 28% of ADPKD patients have symptomatic renal stone disease; this incidence is approximately 7- to 10-fold higher than the incidence in the general population [3,4]. In one study, 36% of individuals with ADPKD were found on computed tomography (CT) imaging to have renal stones in absence of any symptoms [5]. Additionally, more than half of the renal stones in this patient population are of uric acid composition in comparison to the other stone formers, where uric acid accounts for 8 to 10% of the calculi. The anatomic abnormalities noted in those with ADPKD add additional challenges to determining the etiology of pain. High complication rates of interventional/surgical management of nephrolithiasis in this population further highlight the importance of preventative medical and dietary therapies to minimize further stone formation. In this chapter we will discuss the various aspects of nephrolithiasis unique to the ADPKD population.

Lithogenic Risk Factors in ADPKD

The overall high incidence of nephrolithiasis, especially the increased occurrence of uric acid stones in those with ADPKD, suggests there are factors intrinsic to this disease that contribute to lithogenesis in this population.

Initially, compression or distortion of the renal collecting system by expanding cysts and resultant urinary stasis were believed to be the primary factors leading to the increased incidence of stones [6]. In a comparative study, Grampsas et al. prospectively evaluated 48 ADPKD patients, 15 of whom were stone formers and 33 non-stone formers. ADPKD patients with nephrolithiasis had a greater number of cysts and a significantly larger predominant cyst size compared with patients without nephrolithiasis; this difference was most pronounced when calculi were noted in only one kidney [7]. Another investigation of 125 individuals with ADPKD identified renal volume of $\geq$ 500 ml to be an independent predictor of subsequent stone formation [8]. In addition to the mechanical factors contributing to stone formation in this population, evaluating the twenty-four hour urine collections can demonstrate metabolic factors that are responsible for frequent occurrence of nephrolithiasis in ADPKD. Individual metabolic risk factors include:

1. Reduced urinary excretion of natural inhibitors of crystallization:

Citrate and magnesium are powerful micro-molecular inhibitors of crystal formation and aggregation in the renal collecting system. Both hypocitraturia and hypomagnesuria are more common in the ADPKD population as compared to the general population. Torres et al. documented hypocitraturia as a risk factor for nephrolithiasis in ADPKD [3]. In a retrospective analysis of 751 ADPKD patients, hypocitraturia and a low urine pH were the most common metabolic alterations. In the above referenced study by Grampsas et al., two consecutive 24 hour urine samples from the patients with ADPKD demonstrated lower daily urinary citrate excretion (309.5 mg/day) irrespective of the presence of nephrolithiasis [7]. While the daily citrate excretion was lower among stone formers (247.3 ± 58.6 mg/day) as compared to ADPKD non-stone formers (337.7 ± 36.9 mg/day), these results did not reach statistical significance. For reference, normal urinary citrate is in the range of 500-550 mg/day.

These results were confirmed by a recent analysis that showed that the daily urinary citrate excretion in 33 ADPKD patients with stones (295 mg/day) was not different from the median value in 90 patients without stones (301 mg/day), although still significantly lower than normal urinary citrate excretion [8]. Whether hypocitraturia represents an abnormality inherent in ADPKD or an acquired derangement as a consequence of progression of renal disease over time is not known.

Similarly, the incidence of hypomagnesuria is increased in ADPKD, whether they are stone formers or not. In the Grampsas study, the mean daily magnesium excretion in the group with nephrolithiasis (64.6 ± 7.2) was lower than in those without nephrolithiasis (92.6 ± 5.5) [7]. A more recent investigation of 125 ADPKD patients noted above found that the incidence of hypomagnesiuria was increased in both groups [8]. The underlying reason for this metabolic derangement is not understood. More recently, chronic proton pump inhibitor (PPI) use has been associated with hypomagnesemia and lower 24-hour urine magnesium excretion [9]. As such, patients using this class of medications may be at increased risk for stone formation. Since ADPKD patients already have low urine magnesium excretion compared to the general population, this patient cohort may be especially vulnerable to the lithogenic effect of PPIs.

2. Increased urinary acid excretion:

The high incidence of uric acid nephrolithiasis that is observed in ADPKD suggests that uric acid metabolism may be altered [10]. However, various studies have shown that uric acid homeostasis is preserved in individuals with ADPKD. Kaehny et al. studied 163 subjects with ADPKD and 138 relatives without ADPKD [11]. Presence of hyperuricemia, uric acid clearance and factional excretion of uric acid did not differ between the subjects in the two groups with normal renal function. Hyperuricemia and deceased renal excretion of uric acid that developed in ADPKD patients with impaired renal function was not different from what was observed in the control population. The propensity for uric acid crystallization in these patients appears to be related to a low urine pH. Multiple studies have shown that a majority of the patients with ADPKD have urine pH less than 5.5 [3, 7, 8, 12].

There is evidence documenting increased activation of the renin-angiotensin-aldosterone-system (RAAS) related to local parenchymal ischemia due to cyst expansion in ADPKD [13-15]. Angiotensin and aldosterone stimulate H+ ATPase activity in the type A acid secreting intercalated cells [16]. This may represent one of the mechanisms responsible for increased urinary acidification observed in ADPKD and therefore, the propensity for uric acid precipitation.

Diagnosis of Nephrolithiasis in ADPKD

Nephrolithiasis should be considered in the differential diagnosis of any patient with ADPKD presenting with acute abdominal or flank pain. Beyond a thorough history that includes details about prior episodes of stone disease, stone composition and any procedures the patient may have had, and a careful physical examination, imaging is needed to confirm the diagnosis. A few comments about choice of imaging modality specific to ADPKD are noteworthy:

- In the non-ADPKD stone former, ultrasonography and abdominal CT imaging are equal in detecting the presence of stones. In contrast, CT imaging is more sensitive than ultrasonography in detecting stones in the PKD population because of the altered renal anatomy caused by cyst formation [8, 17, 18]. However, it should be noted that renal calcifications detected by unenhanced CT scans are seen in nearly half the patients with ADPKD; these can represent either cyst calcifications or renal calculi or a combination of the two [5]. CT performed with and without intravenous contrast enhancement allows differentiation between stones and cyst calcifications, and offers the highest specificity for making the diagnosis of nephrolithiasis. However, use of iodinated contrast is often limited by the risk of contrast-induced nephropathy, especially in presence of acute or chronic renal function impairment. High-resolution CT imaging without contrast is recommended for these patients.
- Radiolucent uric acid stones account for about 50% of the stones in this population. Since they would be missed by a plain abdominal

film, CT imaging should be employed as the preferred radiologic study.

Acute Renal Colic Management in ADPKD

Renal colic due to nephrolithiasis in any patient is due to an increase in intraluminal pressure from ureteric obstruction, stretching the nerve endings in the mucosa and smooth muscle in the wall of the ureter [19]. The ureter contracts as it attempts to push the stone forward; this produces colicky pain. If the stone becomes lodged and is unable to move, the muscles go into a prolonged isotonic contraction. The result is an increased production of lactic acid that irritates both slow-type A and fast-type C fibers. Additionally, as renal pelvic pressure increases, renal blood flow begins to decline. This leads to an auto-regulatory increase in prostaglandin-mediated pre-glomerular vasodilation and increase in renal blood flow (RBF). The RBF increase causes a diuresis, with resultant further increase in renal pelvic pressure and leading to worsening of the pain. Most patients can be managed conservatively with pain medication and hydration until the stone passes. It should be noted that many randomized prospective studies comparing non-steroidal anti-inflammatory drugs (NSAIDs) with morphine suggest that both agents provide comparable pain relief [20,21]. The analgesic effect of NSAIDs is related to both the local anti-inflammatory action and antagonism of the diuretic effect of prostaglandins (via pre-glomerular arteriolar dilation and inhibitory effect on anti-diuretic hormone activity). Because of the known adverse effects of NSAIDs on kidney function, they should be used with caution.We recommend their use be limited to less than 3 days duration, while ensuring patients are volume replete. Monitoring renal function and urine output are necessary when using NSAIDs.

A team approach of nephrologist and urologist is essential in the PKD patient because of the potential risks of urosepsis, acute kidney injury, hydronephrosis and non-passage of stone (leading to unyielding pain). In one study by Torres et al, nearly 20% of the patients with ADPKD and symptomatic nephrolithiasis required urological interventions [3].

The procedure performed in a large majority of these patients two to three decades ago was open surgery (sometimes including nephrectomy). Minimally invasive technology, such as extracorporeal shock wave lithotripsy (ESWL) and percutaneous nephrolithotomy (PCNL), has superseded the use of open surgery for management of stone disease in the general population, and is now being increasingly applied to ADPKD. Evidence regarding efficacy and risks of commonly used endo-urological procedures are discussed below:

1. ESWL:

ESWL is the most common intervention used for stone management, including in the cohort with ADPKD. It has been shown to be successful and safe in multiple case series. In a study published by Delakas in 1997, an average of 1800 shockwaves with low energy (mean 18kV, range 15 to 21 kV) were applied to 16 renal units in 13 patients [22]. Other than transient gross hematuria (not requiring any transfusions), no complications were seen in patients undergoing the procedure. 11 patients (85%) were stone free 3 months after lithotripsy; a second treatment was necessary in only 2 patients. In a follow up study by Ng et al, 4 out of 7 patients requiring urological intervention underwent ESWL, with satisfactory results and no complications in any of the patients [23]. Baishya et al. recently described successful use of ESWL with low energy shocks (less than 13kV; limited to less than 1500 in one sitting) in two patients; no hematuria or pain related to cyst hemorrhage was observed [24].

2. PCNL:

Larger (>20 mm) upper urinary tract stones usually cannot be managed adequately by ESWL alone. Flexible ureteroscopy with a holmium laser may be an option for smaller upper tract stones [25]. For larger or multiple upper urinary tract stones, PCNL is frequently required. However, the narrow and long calyceal spaces seen in ADPKD add to the procedural complexity and complication rate with this procedure. Umbreit and colleagues performed PCNL in 11 kidneys in 9 patients [10]. While two access tracts were necessary in 5 kidneys and a second stage endoscopic procedure with ultrasonic lithotripsy was required in 2 kidneys, complete stone removal was documented using a nephrostogram in 9 (82%) of 11 kidneys. With a mean follow up of 2.7 years, there were no postoperative complications, no deterioration in renal function or recurrent stones. In a study published by Srivastava in 2011, PCNL was done in 25 kidneys among 22 patients with average stone size of 2.4 cm ± 0.8 cm [26]. Complete stone clearance after one-stage procedure was seen in 20 (88%) of 25 kidneys. Two patients had residual fragments of 3 mm each, two patients required relook PCNL for larger residual stone fragments and one required follow-up ESWL. Postoperatively, four patients had fever (including fungemia in one patient), three patients required blood transfusions and none required angio-embolization. Another recent study by Singh et al. showed a similarly high success and low complication rate in a cohort of 22 patients

[27]. Recently, Lei et al. described a modified PCNL technique using a miniaturized scope through a 18F or smaller nephrostomy tract (as opposed to conventional PCNL that utilizes a 24 to 34F renal access tract) in 23 renal units in 23 patients; similar success and low complication rates were observed with their technique [28].

In summary, for ADPKD patients with symptomatic nephrolithiasis where urologic intervention is needed, ESWL is indicated as the first line treatment for stones up to 20 mm in size. For upper urinary tract stones larger than 20 mm and in failed cases of ESWL, PCNL is the preferred modality. The risk of post-operative complications, such as bleeding requiring blood transfusions and fever, as well as the risk of repeat procedures for removal of residual stone fragments, is higher in ADPKD as compared to the general population. As such, all ADPKD patients should be referred to a nephrologist for a comprehensive stone evaluation and detailed recommendations regarding preventative measures to decrease the potential for new stone formation.

Secondary Stone Prevention in ADPKD

As in any other patient with a high propensity for stone formation, the first step in the management of these patients is identification of stone composition and underlying major risk factors:

- Patients should be encouraged to retrieve stones for analysis.
- Examination of the urine sediment for presence of crystals.
- Serum chemistries (including serum calcium and phosphate), uric acid, parathyroid hormone and 25-hydroxy vitamin D measured at initial evaluation to look for systemic metabolic abnormalities that may explain the proclivity towards lithogenesis.
- At least two to three weeks after acute renal or ureteral obstruction is resolved, a 24-hour urine collection should be obtained while the patient maintains their usual diet, fluid intake and physical activity. Measurements should include total volume, pH, uric acid, calcium, phosphorus, oxalate, citrate, magnesium, sodium, ammonium, sulfate, urea nitrogen and calculated protein catabolic rate. To assess completeness of the sample, urine creatinine should be measured as well. Additionally, urinary supersaturation of uric acid, calcium oxalate and calcium phosphate should be calculated. Given the high variability of the urine values, some experts recommend two 24-hour

collections, and a third one if there is substantial discrepancy between the two results.

The general principles of secondary stone prevention apply to the ADPKD population. Aspects of care specific to this-risk population include:

1. Free water intake:

Increased free water intake remains the basic tenet of treatment. Among stone formers, intake of 2.5 L per day is associated with a 29% risk reduction in first stone recurrence [29,30]. In addition to primary and secondary prevention of stone formation, increased water intake may have a beneficial role in reduction of cyst growth, and ultimately preservation of renal function. Vasopressin has been shown to increase cyclic 3'-5'-adenosine monophosphate levels in the epithelium of renal cysts, and lead to cyst growth [31]. In the randomized double-blinded, placebo-controlled TEMPO 3:4 clinical trial of 1445 ADPKD patients with preserved glomerular filtration rate, the vasopressin receptor 2 (V2) antagonist, tolvaptan, was shown to lead to a statistically significant reduction in the annual kidney volume increment (2.8% growth in tolvaptan group vs. 5.5% in placebo group) over three years [32]. Rate of kidney function decline (reciprocal of the serum creatinine level) was significantly slower in the tolvaptan group (-2.61 ml/mg per year) as compared to the placebo group (-3.81 ml/mg per year). An alternative might be to lower ADH concentration by increasing water intake. In a rat model for ADPKD, a 3.5-fold increased water intake reduced renal expression of the V2 receptor, urine osmolality and kidney weight compared with normal water intake [33]. However, these results were not reproduced in the only study done in humans [34]. Due to methodological considerations, beneficial effects of increased fluid intake on renal cyst growth cannot be ruled out. Based on the evidence available, we recommend all patients with ADPKD and stones should maintain a daily fluid intake of at least 2.5 to 3.0 L per day.

2. Citrate and magnesium supplementation:

Potassium citrate supplementation can be useful in management of lithogenic urinary metabolic derangements in ADPKD through two mechanisms: 1) urinary alkalization; 2) increasing urinary citrate concentration. While potassium citrate tablet preparations are available, typically 8 to 12 tablets a day may be needed to achieve adequate urine citrate levels. The large pill burden may affect the compliance in these patients. Alternatively, lemon juice concentrate (which contains potassium citrate) diluted in water has been shown to be an effective alternate [35]. We recommend three to four tablespoons of lemon juice concentrate to a liter of water, and consuming it over the course of the day. This regimen combines both increased fluid intake and citrate intake, and in our experience, patients find it easier to incorporate this into their daily routine than citrate tablets. As noted earlier, magnesium is another powerful inhibitor of stone formation. Oral magnesium supplementation may be necessary if the daily magnesium excretion falls below the reference range of 75 to 150 mg/day [36].

3. **Urinary alkalinization and xanthine oxidase inhibitors for patients with uric acid stones:**

Correcting the low urine pH is the most important modifiable risk factor in patients with uric acid nephrolithiasis. At a urine pH of 6.75 more than 90 percent of the total urinary uric acid is in the form of more soluble urate salt, thereby minimizing the risk of uric acid precipitation. This can be achieved using citrate supplements (as described above) or bicarbonate supplementation.

A urine pH between 6.5 and 7.0 should be the target. It should be noted that alkalization with potassium salts is preferable over sodium citrate or sodium bicarbonate, as the increased sodium load may increase urinary calcium excretion, thereby adding to the risk of calcium stone formation [37]. If patients continue to form uric acid stones despite alkali therapy and increased fluid intake (usually in setting of a high serum uric acid level and hyperuricosuria), chronic administration of a xanthine oxidase inhibitor, such as allopurinol, to lower uric acid production and excretion may be required.

Lastly, as noted earlier in this chapter, an overactive RAAS appears to be one of the mechanisms responsible for increased urinary acidification observed in these patients. Based on this, it can be hypothesized that pharmacologic blockade of the RAAS using angiotensin converting enzyme inhibitors, angiotensin receptor blockers and aldosterone antagonists will block the secretion of H+ in exchange for K+ in the intercalated cells of the cortical collecting tubules.

The two recent publications based on the HALT-PKD trial evaluated the effects of RAAS antagonists in ADPKD [38,39]. A follow-up analysis by the HALT-PKD group will evaluate whether use of these drugs leads to an increase in urine pH. It will be determined if the increase in pH is sufficient to prevent uric acid crystallization as a prelude to recommending these medications in stone management in ADPKD.

4. **Follow-up and patient education:**

As in any other patient with recurrent stone disease, a follow-up 24 hour urine is critical to assess patient compliance, to evaluate effectiveness of administered therapies, and to determine if any changes to the ongoing treatment regimen are needed. Also, it cannot be overemphasized that patient education regarding risk of recurrence and need for long-term (frequently, life-long) management of each individual metabolic risk factor is integral to effective management of these patients.

References

[1] Gabow PA. Autosomal dominant polycystic kidney disease. *N. Engl. J. Med.* 1993 Jul 29;329(5):332–42.

[2] Gabow PA. Autosomal dominant polycystic kidney disease--more than a renal disease. *Am. J. Kidney Dis.* 1990 Nov;16(5):403–13.

[3] Torres VE, Erickson SB, Smith LH, Wilson DM, Hattery RR, Segura JW. The association of nephrolithiasis and autosomal dominant polycystic kidney disease. *Am. J. Kidney Dis.* 1988 Apr;11(4):318–25.

[4] Dimitrakov D, Simeonov S. Studies on nephrolithiasis in patients with autosomal dominant polycystic kidney disease. *Folia Med* (Plovdiv). 1994;36(3):27–30.

[5] Levine E, Grantham JJ. Calcified renal stones and cyst calcifications in autosomal dominant polycystic kidney disease: clinical and CT study in 84 atients. *Am. J. Roentgenol.* 1992 Jul;159(1):77–81.

[6] Amar AD, Das S, Egan RM. Management of urinary calculous disease in patients with renal cysts: review of 12 years of experience in 18 patients. *J. Urol.* 1981 Feb;125(2):153–6.

[7] Grampsas SA, Chandhoke PS, Fan J, Glass MA, Townsend R, Johnson AM, et al. Anatomic and metabolic risk factors for nephrolithiasis in patients with autosomal dominant polycystic kidney disease. *Am. J. Kidney Dis.* 2000 Jul;36(1):53–7.

[8] Nishiura JL, Neves RFCA, Eloi SRM, Cintra SMLF, Ajzen SA, Heilberg IP. Evaluation of nephrolithiasis in autosomal dominant polycystic kidney disease patients. *Clin. J. Am. Soc. Nephrol.* 2009 Apr;4(4):838–44.

[9] William JH, Nelson R, Hayman N, Mukamal KJ, Danziger J. Proton-pump inhibitor use is associated with lower urinary magnesium excretion. *Nephrology* (Carlton). 2014 Dec;19(12):798–801.

[10] Umbreit EC, Childs MA, Patterson DE, Torres VE, LeRoy AJ, Gettman MT. Percutaneous nephrolithotomy for large or multiple upper tract

calculi and autosomal dominant polycystic kidney disease. *J. Urol.* 2010 Jan;183(1):183–7.

[11] Kaehny WD, Tangel DJ, Johnson AM, Kimberling WJ, Schrier RW, Gabow PA. Uric acid handling in autosomal dominant polycystic kidney disease with normal filtration rates. Am. J. Med. 1990 Jul;89(1):49–52.

[12] Torres VE, Wilson DM, Hattery RR, Segura JW. Renal stone disease in autosomal dominant polycystic kidney disease. *Am. J. Kidney Dis.* 1993 Oct;22(4):513–9.

[13] Chapman AB, Stepniakowski K, Rahbari-Oskoui F. Hypertension in autosomal dominant polycystic kidney disease. *Adv. Chronic Kidney Dis.* 2010 Mar;17(2):153–63.

[14] Loghman-Adham M, Soto CE, Inagami T, Cassis L. The intrarenal renin-angiotensin system in autosomal dominant polycystic kidney disease. *Am. J. Physiol. Renal Physiol.* 2004 Oct;287(4):F775–88.

[15] Kocyigit I, Yilmaz MI, Unal A, Ozturk F, Eroglu E, Yazici C, et al. A link between the intrarenal renin angiotensin system and hypertension in autosomal dominant polycystic kidney disease. *Am. J. Nephrol.* 2013;38(3):218–25.

[16] Pech V, Zheng W, Pham TD, Verlander JW, Wall SM. Angiotensin II activates H+-ATPase in type A intercalated cells. *J. Am. Soc. Nephrol.* 2008 Jan;19(1):84–91.

[17] Gupta S, Seith A, Sud K, Kohli HS, Singh SK, Sakhuja V, et al. CT in the evaluation of complicated autosomal dominant polycystic kidney disease. *Acta Radiol.* 2000 May;41(3):280–4.

[18] Lawson TL, McClennan BL, Shirkhoda A. Adult polycystic kidney disease: ultrasonographic and computed tomographic appearance. *J. Clin. Ultrasound.* 1978 Oct;6(5):297–302.

[19] Shokeir AA. Renal colic: new concepts related to pathophysiology, diagnosis and treatment. Curr. Opin. Urol. 2002 Jul;12(4):263–9.

[20] Cordell WH, Larson TA, Lingeman JE, Nelson DR, Woods JR, Burns LB, et al. Indomethacin suppositories versus intravenously titrated morphine for the treatment of ureteral colic. Ann. Emerg. Med. 1994 Feb;23(2):262–9.

[21] Hetherington JW, Philp NH. Diclofenac sodium versus pethidine in acute renal colic. Br. Med. J. (Clin Res Ed). 1986 Jan 25;292(6515):237–8.

[22] Delakas D, Daskalopoulos G, Cranidis A. Extracorporeal shockwave lithotripsy for urinary calculi in autosomal dominant polycystic kidney disease. *J.. Endourol.* 1997 Jun;11(3):167–70.

[23] Ng CS, Yost A, Streem SB. Nephrolithiasis associated with autosomal dominant polycystic kidney disease: contemporary urological management. *J. Urol.* 2000 Mar;163(3):726–9.

[24] Baishya R, Dhawan DR, Kurien A, Ganpule A, Sabnis RB, Desai MR. Management of nephrolithiasis in autosomal dominant polycystic kidney disease - A single center experience. *Urol. Ann.* 2012 Jan;4(1):29–33.

[25] Yili L, Yongzhi L, Ning L, Dongwei X, Chunlai L, Suomin L, et al. Flexible ureteroscopy and holmium laser lithotripsy for treatment of upper urinary tract calculi in patients with autosomal dominant polycystic kidney disease. *Urol. Res.* 2012 Feb;40(1):87–91.

[26] Srivastava A, Bansal R, Srivastava A, Chaturvedi S, Ranjan P, Ansari MS, et al. Percutaneous nephrolithotomy in polycystic kidney disease: is it safe and effective? *Int. Urol. Nephrol.* 2011 Nov 20;44(3):725–30.

[27] Singh V, Sinha RJ, Gupta DK. Percutaneous Nephrolithotomy in autosomal dominant polycystic kidney disease: Is it different from percutaneous nephrolithotomy in normal kidney? *Curr. Urol.* 2013 Aug;7(1):7–13.

[28] Lei M, Zhu W, Wan SP, Liu Y, Zeng G, Yuan J. Safety and efficacy of minimally invasive percutaneous nephrolithotomy in patients with autosomal dominant polycystic kidney disease. *J. Endourol.* 2014 Jan;28(1):17–22.

[29] Taylor EN, Stampfer MJ, Curhan GC. Dietary factors and the risk of incident kidney stones in men: new insights after 14 years of follow-up. *J. Am. Soc. Nephrol.* 2004 Dec;15(12):3225–32.

[30] Curhan GC, Willett WC, Knight EL, Stampfer MJ. Dietary factors and the risk of incident kidney stones in younger women: Nurses' Health Study II. *Arch. Intern. Med.* 2004 Apr 26;164(8):885–91.

[31] Wang X, Wu Y, Ward CJ, Harris PC, Torres VE. Vasopressin directly regulates cyst growth in polycystic kidney disease. *J. Am. Soc. Nephrol.* 2008 Jan;19(1):102–8.

[32] Torres VE, Chapman AB, Devuyst O, Gansevoort RT, Grantham JJ, Higashihara E, et al. Tolvaptan in patients with autosomal dominant polycystic kidney disease. *N. Engl. J. Med.* 2012 Dec 20;367(25):2407–18.

[33] Nagao S, Nishii K, Katsuyama M, Kurahashi H, Marunouchi T, Takahashi H, et al. Increased water intake decreases progression of polycystic kidney disease in the PCK rat. *J. Am. Soc. Nephrol.* 2006 Aug;17(8):2220–7.

[34] Higashihara E, Nutahara K, Tanbo M, Hara H, Miyazaki I, Kobayashi K, et al. Does increased water intake prevent disease progression in autosomal dominant polycystic kidney disease? *Nephrol. Dial. Transplant.* 2014 Sep;29(9):1710–9.

[35] Aras B, Kalfazade N, Tuğcu V, Kemahli E, Ozbay B, Polat H, et al. Can lemon juice be an alternative to potassium citrate in the treatment of urinary calcium stones in patients with hypocitraturia? A prospective randomized study. *Urol. Res.* 2008 Dec;36(6):313–7.

[36] Kato Y, Yamaguchi S, Yachiku S, Nakazono S, Hori J-I, Wada N, et al. Changes in urinary parameters after oral administration of potassium-sodium citrate and magnesium oxide to prevent urolithiasis. *Urology.* 2004 Jan;63(1):7–11–discussion11–2.

[37] Pak CY, Sakhaee K, Fuller C. Successful management of uric acid nephrolithiasis with potassium citrate. *Kidney Int.* 1986 Sep;30(3):422–8.

[38] Schrier RW, Abebe KZ, Perrone RD, Torres VE, Braun WE, Steinman TI, et al. Blood pressure in early autosomal dominant polycystic kidney disease. *N. Engl. J. Med.* 2014 Dec 11;371(24):2255–66.

[39] Torres VE, Abebe KZ, Chapman AB, Schrier RW, Braun WE, Steinman TI, et al. Angiotensin blockade in late autosomal dominant polycystic kidney disease. *N. Engl. J. Med.* 2014 Dec 11;371(24):2267–76.

Index

A

B

C

D

T